MW00534514

PREPARING

FOR A

Gentle Birth

———————

"Women are not often told how amazing their pelvises are, but this fact is extremely evident during the act of giving birth. Blandine Calais-Germain gives us a detailed understanding of the dynamic and cooperative process between the mother and the baby during which the pelvis moves and adjusts. Every millimeter of extra space that the pelvis can provide during this process is essential to a quick and easy birth. Every mother will benefit from learning the simple movements she can practice during pregnancy that help prepare her for giving birth. Every care provider will benefit from gaining a new respect for the simple and effective ways to facilitate the movement of the baby through the pelvis during childbirth. This book will become an essential text for every midwife, doctor, and doula. Calais-Germain illustrates beautifully that if you can't move the baby, simply move the mother and her pelvis."

BARBARA HARPER, R.N., MIDWIFE, DOULA, FOUNDER OF WATERBIRTH INTERNATIONAL, AND AUTHOR OF *GENTLE BIRTH CHOICES*

PREPARING
FOR A
Gentle Birth

The Pelvis in Pregnancy

Blandine Calais-Germain
and Núria Vives Parés

Translated by Martine Curtis Oakes

Healing Arts Press
Rochester, Vermont • Toronto, Canada

Healing Arts Press
One Park Street
Rochester, Vermont 05767
www.HealingArtsPress.com

Healing Arts Press is a division of Inner Traditions International

Copyright © 2009 Éditions DésIris
English translation copyright © 2012 by Inner Traditions International
Originally published in French under the title *Bouger en accouchant* by Éditions DésIris
First U.S. edition published in 2012 by Healing Arts Press

All rights reserved. No part of this book may be reproduced or utilized in any form or by any means, electronic or mechanical, including photocopying, recording, or by any information storage and retrieval system, without permission in writing from the publisher.

Note to the reader: *This book is intended as an informational guide. The remedies, approaches, and techniques described herein are meant to supplement, and not to be a substitute for, professional medical care or treatment. They should not be used to treat a serious ailment without prior consultation with a qualified health care professional.*

Library of Congress Cataloging-in-Publication Data
Calais-Germain, Blandine.
  [Bouger en accouchant. English]
  Preparing for a gentle birth : the pelvis in pregnancy / Blandine Calais-Germain and Núria Vives Parés ; translated by Martine Curtis Oakes. — 1st U.S. ed.
       p. ; cm.
  Originally published in French under the title Bouger en accouchant by Éditions DésIris, c2009.
  Includes bibliographical references and index.
  ISBN 978-1-59477-388-4 (pbk.) — ISBN 978-1-59472-813-1 (e-book)
  1. Childbirth. 2. Labor (Obstetrics) 3. Pelvis. I. Vives Parés, Núria. II. Title.
  [DNLM: 1. Parturition—physiology. 2. Movement—physiology. 3. Pelvis—physiology. WQ 300a]
  RG525.C2813 2011
  618.2—dc23
                                                                        2011025127

Printed and bound in India by Replika Pvt. Ltd.

10   9   8   7   6   5   4   3   2   1

Text design and layout by Virginia Scott Bowman
This book was typeset in Garamond Premier Pro and Gill Sans with Times New Roman,
    Helvetica, and Gill Sans used as display typefaces
Drawings by Blandine Calais-Germain
Graphics by Lauriane Tiberghien

To our mothers, who accompanied us . . .
and whom we have accompanied.

CONTENTS

Testimonials

"Just after the workshop 'The Pelvis and Childbirth,' I worked the night shift at a hospital. A young woman came to give birth, and she let us know that she wanted to have a natural childbirth. . . . She stayed almost the whole time on her hands and knees. I observed silently. I understood exactly what she was doing at all times. By herself, she tried to find all of the asymmetrical possibilities: nutation, contranutation, pronation, supination . . .

"She gave birth to a lovely little girl of 7.7 pounds without an episiotomy or any medication. . . . Incredible!

"I would like to thank you for this experience: being a witness to this birth more than made up for all of the caesarean sections and births that require medical intervention that we are inevitably obliged to participate in."

VIOLETTA NAVIO,
MIDWIFE, ALACANT, SPAIN

"We'd like to thank you for the know-how that you bring to our everyday work; the discovery of the intrinsic movements of the pelvis. This allowed us to give priority to the autonomy of women in labor and to improve the obstetric outcome. For many years our profession ignored that the pelvis is mobile. Incorporating this concept into our practice helped us with very simple things like finding a position that facilitates the descent of the baby and the flexion of the fetus's head: all this by just taking into consideration the movement of the pelvis.

"Position changes, the addition of a pliable support under the sacrum, and also the variety of possible positions on the new birthing bed serve to liberate the pelvis. All of these new strategies and tools have become common practice by our team of midwives; it improves the birth process and the satisfaction of the new mother.

"Our team thanks you for increasing our knowledge. We'd also like to thank you on behalf of our patients who have benefited by this new approach."

THE MIDWIVES OF THE
DR. JOSEP TRUETA UNIVERSITY HOSPITAL OF GIRONA, SPAIN

FOREWORD

In Spain, as elsewhere, our way of understanding and addressing the act of childbirth is always in flux.

Driven by diverse factors, both social and scientific, the purpose of these changes is a search for balance between the quality and security of knowledge and modern-day techniques and the desire of a woman to be an active participant in the birth process. That is why it is necessary to revise the traditional preparations for childbirth by adopting new methods and practices that put the woman in the primary role for her best physical and psychological outcome.

From my point of view, through the perspective of change and innovation, this book makes an important contribution to improving our knowledge of movement in the woman's body in preparation for childbirth. Based on observation of anatomical structures involved in childbirth and rigorous analysis, the focus of the authors is to give women (and couples) power over their own bodies and, at the same time, to offer an individual approach for every birthing experience.

This book, *Preparing for a Gentle Birth,* is the continuation of the work and research that Blandine Calais-Germain and Núria Vives Parés have been doing for several years.

Calais-Germain began her educational programs in 1980, culminating in the 1984 release of *Anatomy of Movement,* her central work, which went on to be published in eleven languages and has become a reference book for students of medicine, sports, dance, physical therapy, and other movement modalities. She has since published five complementary works based on movement as it relates to anatomy. In this book, *Preparing for a Gentle Birth,* she has collaborated with Núria Vives Parés, a teacher and psychomotrician who specializes in the instruction of sensory awareness, to develop methods for preparing for childbirth, reeducating the perineum, and preparing for menopause. These methods offer health care practitioners, especially midwives and massage therapists, the opportunity to reorient their work in the direction of active and creative teaching, which can be adapted for every woman.

It is in this spirit of harmony that this publication, *Preparing for a Gentle Birth,* is immersed in the pool of knowledge of the essential structure of childbirth: the pelvis. In this book you will learn about the mobility of the pelvis and why and how this mobility transforms the interior shape during the passage of the fetus.

Using this as a starting point, the book describes different positions and analyzes them in detail, and the reader will learn physical practices that can help prepare the pelvis for the chosen method of childbirth. Numerous drawings of each concept and physical detail are included to aid comprehension. The authors ask the reader to observe the representations of the pelvis and imagine it in movement. This is one of the most important challenges.

In summary, this book holds a significant place in the training of many health professionals who assist women throughout pregnancy and delivery. It is a useful tool that will promote and bring about anticipated changes.

CARMEN BARONA VILAR,
CHIEF OF THE DEPARTMENT OF PERINATAL HEALTH AND PHYSICIAN IN CHARGE
OF LOW-RISK CHILDBIRTH STRATEGIES FOR THE VALENCIA REGION
VALENCIA, SPAIN

A NOTE TO DOCTORS, MIDWIVES, AND MOTHERS

Preparing for a Gentle Birth is not intended exclusively for those in the medical and paramedical professions; it is written for anyone who would like a better understanding of how the pelvis changes during childbirth. This may include pregnant women, anyone preparing to be of assistance during a woman's labor, or anyone who is helping a woman prepare for labor.

We have chosen to use certain laymen's terms in this book to allow it to remain accessible to as many readers as possible. For example, we often use the word *belly* to designate the abdomen. And we've chosen expressions such as *lie down on your back* or *lie down on your side* over *dorsal* or *lateral decubitus*. We have preserved international anatomical nomenclature when it is accessible. When it is not, we have chosen to use the word that is in current usage. For example, we use *iliac bone* in place of *coxal bone*.

This book covers eutocic deliveries (see description on page 41). This type of delivery assumes that the baby will present head first.

What This Book Does Not Cover

The book targets specifically the pelvis as it relates to the passage of the fetus and the movement that childbirth engenders. It does not cover movements of the pelvis with reference to the standing posture (weight distribution, curves . . .) or micromovements of the sacroiliac or restrictions caused by them.

We will not take an in-depth look at the pelvis as a site of the viscera, except to lightly touch on the abdominal organs of the lesser pelvis, or pelvis minor. In order to simplify the presentation, we do not cover the pelvic floor to any great extent.

While this book covers many pathologies or dystocia, it does not deal specifically with pathologies of the pelvis or diseases related to childbirth.

We present a variety of birthing positions, but the analysis of these positions focuses on how they affect the mobility of the pelvis. For the sake of simplification, we do not examine other important ramifications of these positions, such as their impact on respiration, on vascular compression, or on the relationship between the uterus and the diaphragm.

Attention!

All of the movements and manipulations presented in this book are descriptive and for the purpose of movement analysis. Those who undertake these movements and manipulations do so at their own risk.

HOW TO USE THIS BOOK

You can choose chapters according to your interests.

- Start with the anatomy of the pelvis (p. 2)
- Follow the description of pelvic movements (p. 42)
- Learn why and how these movements alter the pelvis (pp. 82 and 145)
- Learn each position in detail (p. 108)
- Practice the movements to prepare the pelvis for childbirth (p. 154)

Throughout the book you will be invited to experiment on your own anatomy.

Boxed areas with the following icon ● indicate how to locate various parts of your body's anatomy

There are also many drawings of magined internal anatomy from participants in my workshops.

All of the drawings in this book are the sole property of the author, Blandine Calais-Germain, and cannot be used or reproduced outside of the context for which they were created without formal authorization. Workbooks with many of these drawings may be ordered (see pp. 167–69).

Testimonials

"I realize that the methods I am teaching, starting with workshops, are the fundamentals for women giving birth: the knowledge of her own pelvis (palpation of her pubic symphysis, ischial tuberosities, iliac crest, and ilium). Observing that the pelvis is not fixed, knowing the positions where it is most free, and knowing how to modify the birth canal . . . these are precious tools that the woman will have at her disposal. I have seen how the birthing mothers become more conscious of their bodies and take more responsibility for their labors."

IRENES SAYAS,
MIDWIFE, ALACANT HEALTH CENTER,
VALENCIA, SPAIN

"From all that I've learned during the workshop 'The Pelvis and Childbirth' with Núria Vives, I use three key ideas in my daily practice as birthing assistant.

"First idea:

"I invite the woman, whether the birth is spontaneous or induced, to get out of bed and do some pelvic movements during a contraction, and then to rest when the contraction is over.

"I've observed less anxiety and more pain tolerance, and better cervical dilation. After a certain period of time, she will want to go back to the bed.

"Second idea:

"I try to put the pelvis in asymmetrical positions. This is possible even with women who have epidurals or who would rather remain in bed. I propose all the variations (flexion, extension, rotation of the legs) to augment both the anterior/posterior and the lateral dimensions of the birth canal. All this aids the progression of the baby's head.

"Third idea:

"For enlarging the transversal diameter when the head tries to cross the third plane between the sciatic spine, I've found it very helpful to have the woman lie on her side with her thigh in abduction and internal rotation. The woman can stay in this position for almost an hour thanks to articulated beds, until the head passes the third plane. After, I propose that she lie on her back for the crowning.

"This practice is very useful in normal deliveries or when there is not a disproportionate size difference between the fetal head and the mother's pelvis, or when there is no fetal distress, or other dystocia that requires medical intervention."

MARIA FERNANDEZ ALCAIDE,
MIDWIFE, LA PAZ UNIVERSITY HOSPITAL,
MADRID, SPAIN

INTRODUCTION

The Pelvis in Motion

During childbirth the head of the fetus changes shape slightly to adapt to the size and shape of the mother's pelvis. This is possible because the bones of the fetus's head are still malleable. Later, the head will slowly return to its initial shape.

The mother's pelvis is much more rigid than the bones of the baby's head. However, small movements between the bones that make up the pelvis are possible. These movements are produced at the level of the pelvic articulations, and they produce a change in the shape of the pelvis. Such a change happens most profoundly in the pelvic area through which the fetus passes, the area called the pelvic cavity.

In the hours preceeding childbirth, the malleability of the pelvis is augmented by the presence of the hormone that makes the ligaments more supple. During the birth, the mother's pelvis can adapt to accommodate the baby's head. This capacity is minimal, but very exact: precisely at this moment every millimeter gained makes the baby's passage easier. The process is a bit like fitting a key into a lock.

The most important thing to understand at this point is that the pelvis moves, and it is capable of changing its internal shape. To promote rather than inhibit this movement on the day of childbirth, we recommend certain positions of the body, and specifically positions of the legs and spine. Furthermore, *women can work on this pelvic mobility* throughout their entire pregnancy.

Numerous witnesses confirm the usefulness of this approach for normal childbirth situations as well as certain dystocia. We will explain why it is common to hear women and midwives say things like "the baby delivered itself" after experiencing the different ways of positioning the spine and legs.

This book describes the dynamic anatomy of the pelvis. It details the movements of the different phases of childbirth and the most effective ways to facilitate them. We will give a selection of positions, attitudes, and postures, and we will explain their effects on the pelvis. Finally, we will offer movements a woman can practice during the pregnancy that will prepare her for the actual birth.

This book speaks, therefore, of the *pelvis in motion,* highlights the fact that the pelvis is malleable on the day of childbirth, and demonstrates that there are movements that favor this malleability. We will present the arguments that support the idea that movement can dramatically help women through labor.

This book will also attest to the profound knowledge that all women inherently possess when bringing a child into the world.

1

WHAT IS THE PELVIS, AND WHAT DOES IT DO?

Our description of the pelvis is not complete but targeted. It is intended to explain the way in which the pelvis moves and changes shape during childbirth. At this time the woman's pelvis is touched, mobilized, pushed, and pulled.

There are some important landmarks to know, such as the places from which we can influence the shape of the pelvis. But the fetus crosses the pelvis in certain internal areas, and though these areas change shape to adapt, for the most part we cannot touch them.

THE GENERAL FORM OF THE PELVIS

The Bony Pelvis

At the union of the trunk and the lower extremities (the legs), the pelvis is like a large bony ring with irregular contours.

On the inside, the pelvis looks like a basin or bowl without a bottom. The "bowl" holds the abdominal viscera. On the outside, the pelvis serves, above all, as a joint for the femurs at the hips. This area is called the *exopelvic surface*.

The pelvis is made up of four bones:

- The **two iliac bones,** situated in the front, on the sides, and even a bit in the back
- The **sacrum,** situated in the back and in the middle
- The **coccyx,** which extends the sacrum toward the lower part of the pelvis

The sacrum and the coccyx are part of the vertebral column (the spine). The two iliac bones belong with the lower extremities.

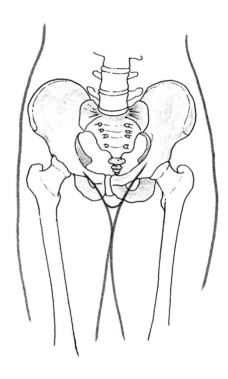

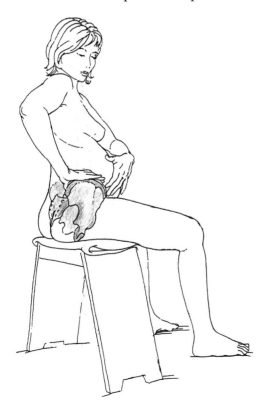

Locate on Yourself

The Totality of the Pelvis

To get a rough idea of the volume of your own pelvis, you can feel it with your hands. The area that is easiest to find is the highest part: the iliac crest. You can also feel for the lowest region: the two ischial tuberosities. The anterior part of the pelvis, the pubic symphysis, joins the two iliac bones. And the posterior part, the sacrum, continues lower to form the coccyx.

How We Imagine the Pelvis

Presenting the pelvis might seem superfluous to the professional obstetrician, and off-putting for some women who will read this book in preparation for childbirth. Is it really useful to describe again the structure of the pelvis? We think it is.

For fifteen years, at the beginning of our workshop sessions, we have asked our participants to draw a picture of a pelvis on a blank piece of paper without a model. We have assembled more than eight hundred drawings, almost all of which were done by those having studied the anatomy of the pelvis. Despite the talent of the artist, which we were not concerned with, we concluded that the shape of the pelvis was not well understood— even by those who work daily with this area of the body. We saw that sometimes parts were even omitted. And in some cases it was impossible to imagine the passage of the fetus through the pelvis, or even the movement of its bones.

Often we proposed that participants do another drawing at the end of the workshop, after having seen and touched the model and having felt, palpated, moved, and recognized their own pelvis. The results would speak for themselves.

We received testimonials from the same professionals telling us how a better understanding of the pelvis profoundly transformed their practice.

We have organized the drawings by theme. Throughout these pages you will find, under the heading "How It's Imagined," text and drawings that illustrate these first attempts.

We thank all of those participants who left the workshop and forgot their drawings, which were still attached to the wall. These drawings have given us the visual documentation for the subject of this book.

How It's Imagined

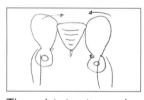 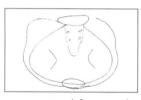 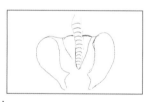

The pelvis in pieces: the parts separated from each other

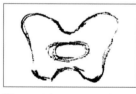 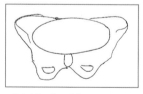 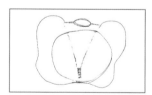

The pelvis as one piece: a solid block of bone

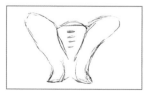 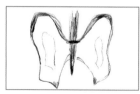 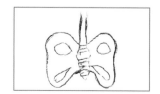

The flat pelvis: like a one-dimensional butterfly

What Does the Iliac Bone Look Like?

It is not easy to make a representation of this bone. It is flat but torqued, which allows it to form the front, sides, and part of the back of each side of the pelvis. It makes up the largest part of the pelvis, and it constitutes, at the same time, both the apex and the base of the pelvis.

Each iliac bone has two surfaces: the external and the internal.

The external surface corresponds primarily to what we think of as the hip.

- Here we find an articular surface in the form of a cup-shaped cavity designed to receive the head of the femur; this is the **(1)** acetabulum, detailed on page 27.
- Above the acetabulum is the area called the **(2)** external iliac fossa.
- Below the acetabulum is a recessed area called the **(3)** obturator foramen. The obturator foramen is bordered:

    From behind by the region of the **(4)** ischium

    From below by the **(5)** ischio-pubic ramus

    In front by the **(6)** pubis

The deep internal endopelvic surface corresponds to the interior of the pelvis.

- In the middle we find an oblique, curved crest: the **(7)** iliopectineal line.
- Above this line is the **(8)** internal iliac fossa.
- Below this line is the bone surrounding the obturator foramen.
- Above and behind the iliopectineal line we find an articular surface in the shape of an "L": the **(9)** auricular surface. This forms a part of the sacroiliac joint, covered in detail on page 19.

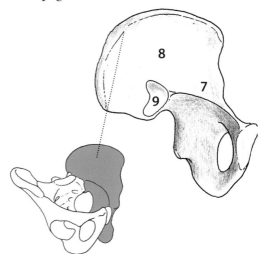

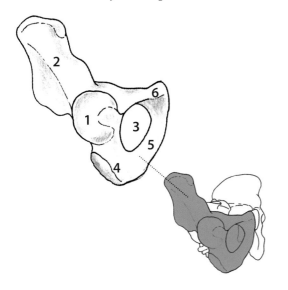

Locate on Yourself

When we mobilize the pelvis, we often have our hands on one part or another of the iliac bone. Likewise, we are often supported by one area or another of this bone.

The Iliac Crest

On the periphery of each iliac bone, we find important landmarks for the subject of this book. The top border, the **(1)** iliac crest, is very easy to palpate.

The farthest forward and often protruding part of the iliac bone is the **(2)** anterior superior iliac spine (ASIS).

The most posterior and less protruding part is the **(3)** posterior superior iliac spine (PSIS).

At the junction between the anterior third and the posterior two-thirds of the iliac crest we find a thickened ridge on the external border: **(4)** the tubercle of the iliac crest.

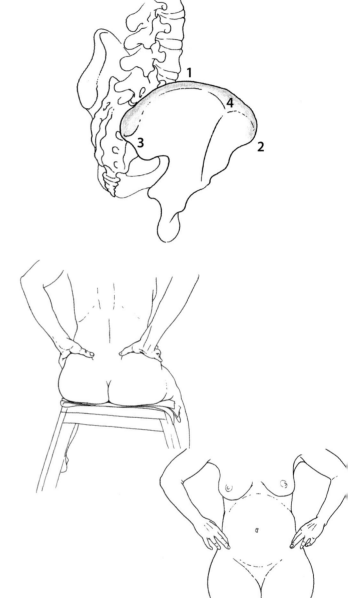

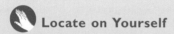

Locate on Yourself

The Iliac Crest and Its Projections

Let your fingers travel the length of the iliac crest. Start in front on the ASIS, which is easy to feel, and take the bony path in different directions: First go up and to the sides, then travel posteriorly and toward the middle of the back. Finish your journey at the PSIS, which is more difficult to find. Along the way try to locate the tubercle of the iliac crest, behind the ASIS.

How It's Imagined

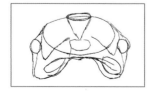 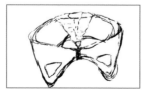 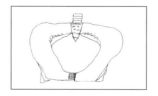

The pelvis without the iliac crest: the sacrum at the same level as the iliac crest

The Front and Back of the Iliac Bone

The Front of the Iliac Bone

It is not easy to palpate the anterior border of the iliac bone because it is crossed by muscles, vessels, and nerves. Here we find the nonpalpable **(1)** anterior inferior iliac spine (AIIS).

The lowest part of this border is the **(2)** pubis. The two iliac bones join at the front of the pubis, forming a joint called the pubic symphysis (detailed on p. 22).

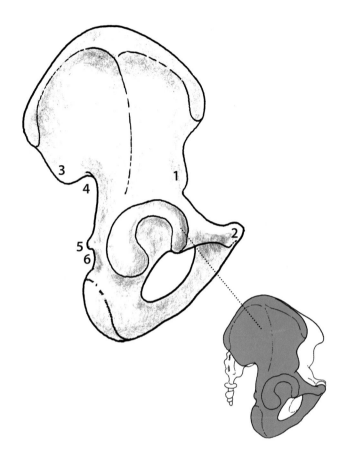

The Back of the Iliac Bone

From top to bottom, the posterior border of the iliac bone is a series of hollows and protrusions, specifically:

- The **(3)** posterior inferior iliac spine
- The **(4)** greater sciatic notch
- The **(5)** ischial spine, projecting inward and to the back
- The **(6)** lesser sciatic notch, descending to the ischium

These last three landmarks elude palpation.

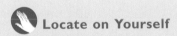 **Locate on Yourself**

The Pubic Symphysis

Just behind the pubic hair, you can feel the width of the area where the two iliac bones meet, with fibrocartilage in the middle. This is the pubic symphysis. Moving toward the abdomen, judge its height as you palpate its superior border, and palpate its inferior border as you move toward the vulva (gently, because in the middle you will find the clitoris).

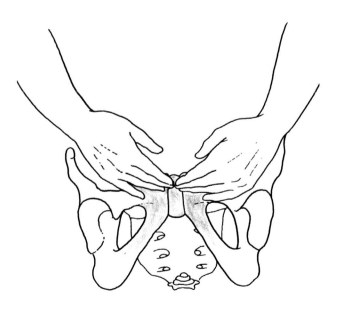

The Ischial Spine (Back of the Iliac Bone)

The ischial spine is a bony eminence found about 4 cm above the ischium.

It is the site of attachment for strong ligaments that connect the iliac bone to the sacrum (see p. 20).

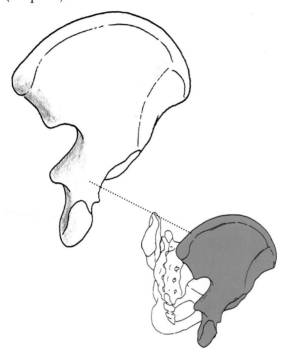

The Orientation of the Ischial Spine

- When the pelvis is viewed in profile, we see that the ischial spine is directed backward.
- When the pelvis is viewed from behind, we see that the ischial spine is directed medially.

The ischial spines make up part of the border of the middle opening of the pelvis. These bony protrusions are very important at the time of delivery: if they are too prominent or point inward too much, they can inhibit the passage of the fetus (see p. 35).

Certain movements of the pelvis, particularly those that move the iliac bones, allow them to change their orientation or the distance between the two ischial spines.

How It's Imagined

In the workshops, after palpating the ischium, participants are often surprised to discover that the ischial spine is very close to the ischium, just above it. We can see here that the ischial spines are drawn on the inside of the pelvis far from the ischium.

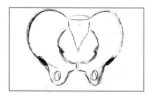
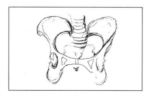
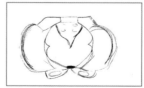

The ischial spines far from the ischium

The Ischium (Bottom of the Iliac Bone)

This investigation of the ischium is fundamental to the recognition of some of the movements of the pelvis talked about later in this book.

The ischium, the lower and posterior part of the iliac bone, is thick and angular.

At the back the ischium, the bone is thick: it is the **ischial tuberosity.** The hamstrings attach here.

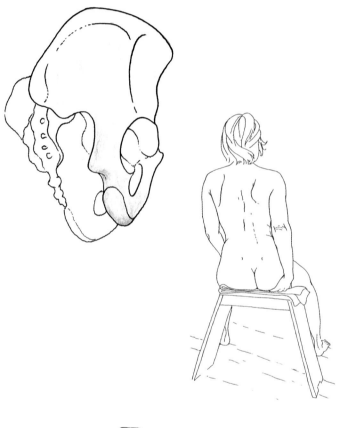

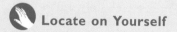 **Locate on Yourself**

The Ischiums

The iliac bone takes a completely different shape at the lower end: it is a tuberosity, large and rounded, coming to a point in the buttocks. In a seated position, you can find the iliac tuberosity by placing your palm or your fingers under one buttock and gradually pressing your weight into the chair. But to better explore this region, you should lie on your side. For example, you can find the left ischial tuberosity while lying on your right side. Bring your left thigh a bit to the front, and run your left hand down the side of your thigh to your buttock, until you find the rounded point of the tuberosity.

If you palpate forward of the ischial tuberosity, you'll arrive at the ischio-pubic ramus. Behind it, the ischium is massive and covered by the buttock. Moving inward, you will locate the region of the perineum, and moving outward, you approach the hip joint.

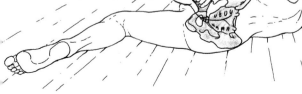

How It's Imagined

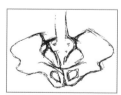 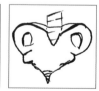

A pelvis without the ischiums

The Ischium and the Iliac Crest Are Part of the Same Iliac Bone

In profile, the iliac bone is shaped like a rectangular plate.

The four corners of the rectangle are prominent physical features.

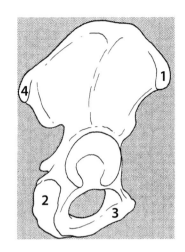

- At the front on the top: **(1)** the anterior superior iliac spine (ASIS)
- At the front on the bottom: **(2)** the pubis
- At the rear on the bottom: **(3)** the ischium
- At the rear on the top: **(4)** the posterior superior iliac spine (PSIS)

In a seated position, the rectangle of the iliac bone is positioned on one of its corners: the one that represents the point of the ischium. Viewed from the front, or a three-quarter view, the rectangle appears to bend in on itself on the diagonal, creating two triangles:

- At the bottom, a triangle facing forward
- At the top, a triangle facing backward

The diagonal bend runs from the ASIS to the ischium, passing by the cotyle, also known as the acetabulum (see p. 27). This is important to understand, because it explains why certain movements that are initiated at the ischium will have an effect on the ASIS and vice versa (see pp. 86–89, and 106).

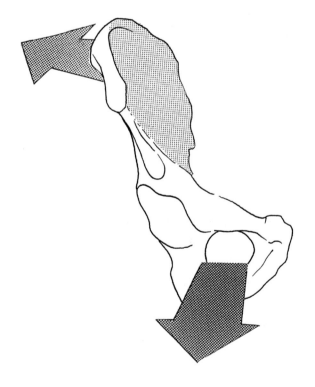

Locate on Yourself

The Ischium–Iliac Crest Relationship

In a seated position, place your right hand under your right buttock where the ischium is most prominent. Place your left hand on the iliac crest on the right side. When you rock your pelvis, you will be able to perceive the movement of the iliac bone between your hands. And, moreover, you will be able to feel that it is a single bone that is moving. However, the upper part and lower parts move in opposite directions.

- If the iliac crest moves forward, the ischium moves backward, and vice versa.
- If the ischiums move apart (the distance is very slight), the iliac crests move toward each other, and vice versa. (It's easiest to feel this movement while lying on your back with your knees bent.)

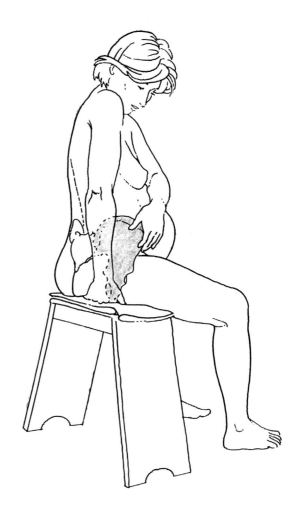

How It's Imagined

We see this confusion in drawings where the iliac crest is drawn separate from the ischium.

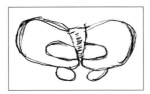 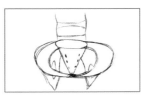 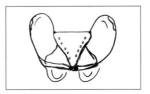

The iliac crest and the ischium as two different bones

The Ischio-Pubic Ramus

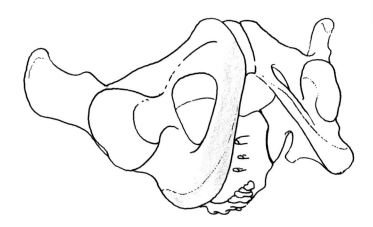

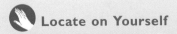
The Ischio-Pubic Ramus

Lie down on your left side. Place your left hand on the right side of the pubic symphysis, and bring your right hand around the back of the thigh to the ischium on the right side. Feel with your fingers for the bony path that joins the two. This ridge of bone is the ischio-pubic ramus. (It is important to the purpose of this book that all women can locate this part of the pelvis on their own body.)

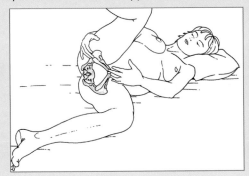

At the bottom of the pelvis, the ischium and pubis are joined by a rather thin band of bone: **the ischio-pubic ramus.**

It runs at an oblique angle to the rest of the iliac bone. It is oblique to the front, top, and middle.

How It's Imagined

Many drawings, like the three shown here, show a horizontal symphysis and the two rami almost parallel.

Some pelvises are missing their anterior parts. They lack the two rami and the ischia.

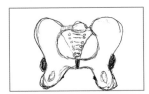
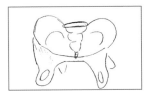
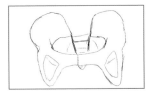

The ischio-pubic ramus far from the pubis

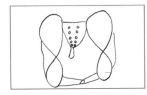
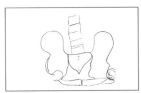
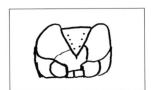

A pelvis without the anterior triangle of the perineum

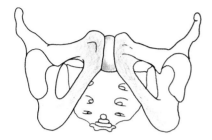

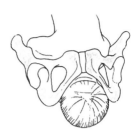

At the bottom of the pelvis, the iliac bones form the opening that the baby passes through. The two pubic rami join in the front, at the pubic symphysis, and form an arch that resembles the vault of a gothic cathedral. It is called the **pelvic outlet.**

This area is fundamental to the subject of this book; it is through here that the baby passes at the last moments of delivery. The angle of this opening varies from one woman to another.

- The more closed or narrow the pelvic outlet is (rather like a masculine pelvis), the more difficult the passage of the baby.
- The more open or wide the outlet is (more like the typical female pelvis), the easier the passage of the baby.

The angle of the outlet can be slightly modified because it includes a malleable part: the fibro-cartilage of the symphysis (see p. 23). This is one of the most important areas where the pelvis can adapt to the passage of the fetal head. In this book (specifically chapter 5), we will see how we can modify the form of this opening more or less symmetrically.

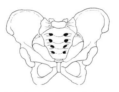

Wide outlet of the female pelvis

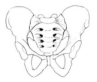

Narrow outlet of the male pelvis

 Locate on Yourself

Outlet of the Anterior Pelvis

Lie on your back with your knees bent and your feet separated. Place a cushion under your buttocks to lift the pelvis and make palpation easier. The pelvis will be slightly tucked, which will make it easier for you to feel the outlet. Start with your hands above the pubic symphysis on the mons pubis, an area that is soft, thick, and sensitive. In its depths you can distinguish the bifurcation of the two ischio-pubic rami that take your hands in opposite directions. Palpate with the fingers of each hand down along the border of each pubic rami, and you will discover two oblique flattened arches, more or less symmetrical, that stretch outward and toward the back of your body until reaching the ischium. During this palpation imagine a triangular window, called the **anterior triangle of the** **perineum,** through which the baby's head will pass. This palpation is very important to the understanding of what follows in this book.

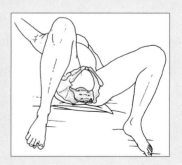

The Sacrum

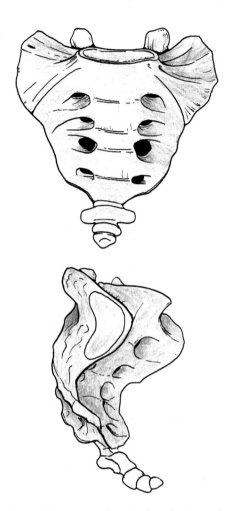

The degree of convexity and concavity varies a lot from one woman to another. These two surfaces, posterior and anterior, are not parallel because the sacrum is thicker at the top (upper third) than at the bottom (lower two-thirds).

This large bone at the back of the pelvis is formed by five vertebrae that have fused but whose vertebral form is still recognizable. Globally, the sacrum has a triangular shape with two surfaces.

- A posterior surface, rather curved (convex), that easily fits the concave form of the palm of the hand and is about the same size
- An anterior surface, convex in shape, that forms the posterior curve of the pelvis (see p. 39) and is the path that the fetal head follows as it descends

Locate on Yourself

The Posterior Surface of the Sacrum

Sit on a stool, or lie down on your side with your knees bent. Put your palm against the back of your pelvis and feel how the shape of the hand adapts to the shape of the sacrum. The tip of the middle finger should be placed at the top of the groove between the buttocks. This is where the lowest part of the sacrum and the upper part of the coccyx meet. You're at the sacrococcygeal symphysis. The heel of your hand is more or less aligned with the top of the sacrum at the sacrolumbar joint. Try to direct the movement of the pelvis using the pressure of your hand, feeling the union of the hand and the pelvis.

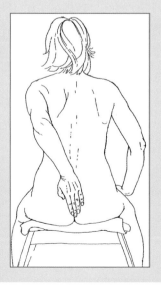

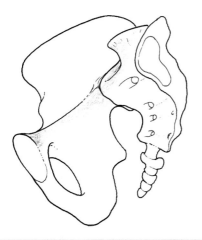

In this book, when we talk about the position of the sacrum in relation to the stages of childbirth, we divide the sacrum into three parts, easily recognizable on the posterior surface.

- "Sacrolumbar" describes the upper area that is connected to the lumbar spine.
- "Middle sacrum" is the middle level, a bit lower than the midline.
- "Sacrococcyx" describes the lower level that touches the coccyx.

When a woman is lying on her back, the pelvis is in a position that allows the fetal head, once it has passed the sacral promontory, to descend to the second third of the sacrum, which is often very concave. The head is then at the area of the posterior perineum, ready to move toward the anterior triangle of the pelvic outlet.

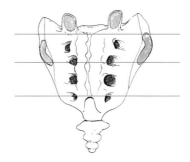

How It's Imagined

Some of the depictions show a pelvis without a sacroiliac joint. The sacrum is at the same height as the iliac crest (top picture at left), or the back of the pelvis is like a solid block (top pictures at center and right).

In some drawings, we see the spinal column pass the pelvis between the two iliac bones, all the way to the coccyx. The sacrum is not represented.

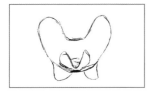 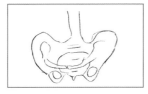 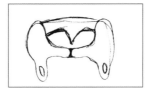

The sacrum and the iliac as a single bone or on the same plane

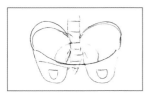 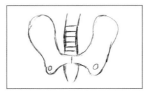 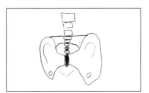

The spine continues to the coccyx

The anterior and posterior surfaces at the top of the sacrum define the limit of the central **(1)** sacral plateau that supports the lowest intervertebral disks (see pp. 25–26).

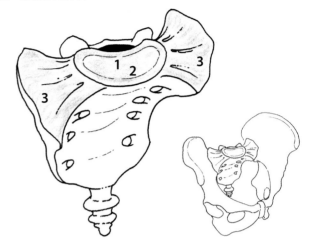

The anterior border of this plateau, called the **(2)** promontory, overlooks the back of the lesser pelvis. This physical location is fundamental to the subject of this book.

On each side of the sacral plateau we find a slightly curved area: the **(3)** sacral wing (or ala sacralis).

It is important to represent this area of the sacrum accurately, with its convex form (promontory) and concave form (sacral wings). When the fetal head passes through this area, it turns toward the hollow of the sacral wings.

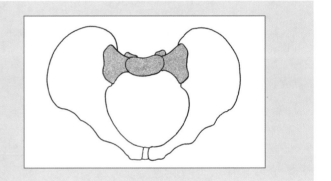

The sacral wings continue along the iliac bone beyond the sacrum along the **(4)** innominate line, forming the lateral and posterior part of the pelvic outlet (see p. 34).

The position of the sacrum can substantially change the orientation of this region (see pp. 46 and 50), a detail that is also fundamental to the subject of this book.

At the bottom, the pointed part of the sacrum articulates with the coccyx.

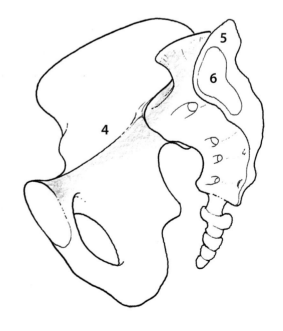

The sacrum also has two lateral borders, which are thicker at the **(5)** top than at the bottom. At the top of each we find a cartilaginous surface that articulates with the iliac **(6)** bone (see "The Sacroiliac Joints," p. 19).

The Coccyx

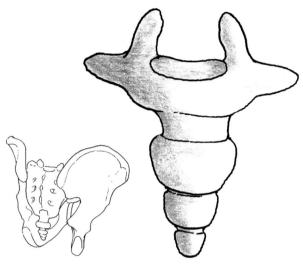

Locate on Yourself

To easily find the coccyx with your hand, lie down on your side with your knees bent. Place your hand over the sacrum (see p. 15). With your middle finger you will feel the top of the coccyx at the top of the groove between your buttocks. Feel its form. Bring your fingers down along one side of the coccyx and then the other so that you get a sense of its two borders. At the end of the coccyx, palpate the rounded part down to the pointed end that is connected to the sphincter of the anus by a small ligament.

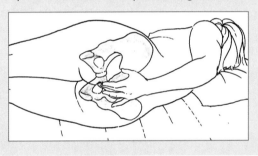

The coccyx is a small bone under the sacrum. It is formed by three to five fused, narrowed vertebrae (although they are not recognizable as vertebrae). An area between the top of the coccyx and the bottom of the sacrum articulates; however, this area tends to ossify after the age of twenty.

Sometimes a woman has an asymmetrical coccyx or one that is pointed downward or internally. This can result from a trauma, from a fall, or following childbirth. This detail becomes particularly important during delivery. However, it is not directly related to the movements described in this work (except that with this position of the coccyx the effects of some movements might be intensified). It is important to know the shape of your own coccyx so that you can choose and modify the positions accordingly (see p. 48). (Modifying the positions to accommodate an asymmetrical coccyx can reduce the pain of childbirth or, if you have an epidural, help you avoid the back pain that sometimes follows the procedure.)

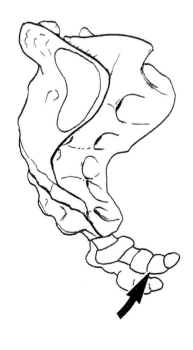

THE BONES OF THE PELVIS
ARTICULATE WITH ONE ANOTHER

Between the three large bones of the pelvis, we find three joints.

- The two sacroiliac joints at the back
- The pubic symphysis at the front

These joints connect the bones of the pelvis and are called *the intrapelvic joints*.

The pelvis also articulates with its neighboring skeletal components.

- The sacrum articulates with the lowest vertebra (L5).

- Each iliac bone articulates with a femur, making up the hips.

These articulations with bones outside of the pelvis are the *extrinsic joints*.

We need to distinguish between these two sorts of joints to avoid confusing the movements of one kind with the movements of the other.

The goal of this work is to mobilize not the joints around the pelvis but the pelvis itself.

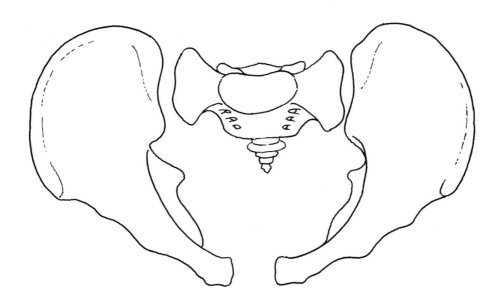

The Sacroiliac Joints

Each iliac bone articulates with a border of the sacrum. These sacroiliac joints unite the cartilaginous surfaces, held in place by a fibrous sleeve: the joint capsule, which is itself reinforced by the ligaments.

The articulating surfaces of the two bones have a similar form.

On the Sacrum

The articulating surface on the sacrum, **(1)** situated on its external border, is a reversed "L" shape and is a bit concave. Where the two arms of the "L" meet, the articulating surface is oval and concave. This detail is important for understanding the variety of movements of the sacroiliac.

On the Iliac Bone

The area of articulation is on the internal surface of the iliac bone, above and behind the **(2)** innominate line. It too is shaped like a reversed "L," but it is a bit convex. Where the two arms of the "L" meet, something of a condyle is formed, that is to say, it is oval and convex. This point too is important for understanding the movements of the sacroiliac.

The Capsule

The capsule is a fibrous sleeve that surrounds the articulating surfaces on each of the two bones. It is thick and transforms the point of articulation into something of a "room," albeit a very small one. This "room" contains a small amount of synovial fluid, which nourishes the cartilage and at the same time lubricates the joint, even though the joint has very limited mobility.

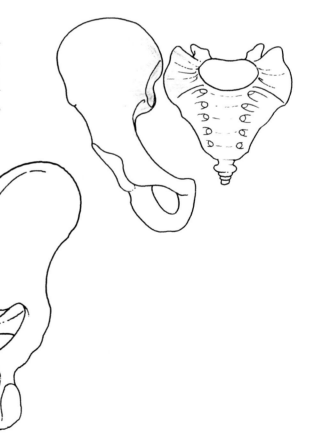

The Many Ligaments around the Sacroiliac Joint

This book does not discuss the role of the ligaments in a static standing posture. We look only at how they pull on the bones of the pelvis, and for that reason we do not describe all of the ligaments.

The ligaments around the sacroiliac joint are numerous and powerful, because they are subjected to a lot of stress when we are in a static standing position.

At the Back

Five **(1)** posterior sacroiliac ligaments link the tuberosities at the back of the sacrum to the internal surface of the iliac bone, behind the area of articulation. These ligaments tend to stop with the movements of contranutation (see p. 50).

At the Bottom, at a Distance from the Joint

- The **(2)** sacrotuberous ligament runs from the lower part of the sacrum and coccyx to the ischium.
- The **(3)** sacrospinous ligament (small or anterior sacrosciatic ligament) runs from the lower sacrum to the ischial spine.

These two ligaments tend to brake nutation (see p. 46).

All of these ligaments are particularly sensitive (see p. 41).

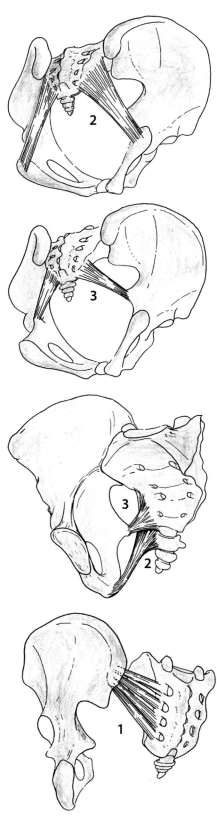

20

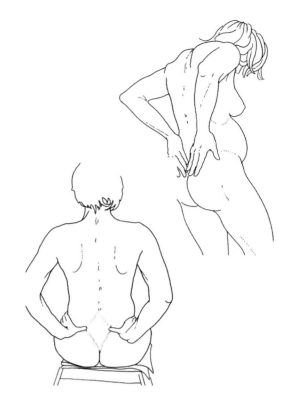

Locate on Yourself

How Can We Explore the Sacroiliac Joints?

The sacroiliac joints are difficult to find on your own body. When a woman is giving birth this is one of the most sensitive and painful areas, because the fetal head pressing against the sacrum puts a lot of stress on the ligaments. Sometimes she will ask for pressure, heat, or simply the contact of a hand to be applied from the outside.

It is therefore important to locate the sacroiliac joints, possibly on someone else. To do this, we look at **Michaelis's rhomboid** (a term used in obstetrics), on the posterior surface of the pelvis at the top of the intergluteal cleft.

The rhomboid is formed, from top to bottom, by:

- The spinous process of L4
- The two PSIS, recognizable by the two dimples they form
- The top of the buttocks

When we are between the two PSIS we are at the sacrolumbar junction (see pp. 25–26).

Above this point a small indentation corresponds to the spinous process of L5; the convex area below corresponds to the sacrum.

It is sometimes painful in the slightly domed areas adjacent to the two PSIS.

Inside the spiny processes are two dimples that mark the location of the sacroiliac joint (they are more or less noticeable depending on the morphology of the woman and whether the sacrum is in nutation or not).

How It's Imagined

The back of the pelvis appears to be a solid block of bone. This region seems to be fixed, without movement between the iliac bone and the sacrum.

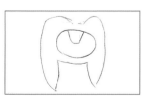 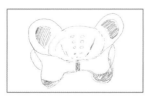 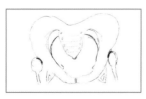

The pelvis without sacroiliac joints

The Pubic Symphysis

At the front of the pelvis the right and left iliac bones are united at the pubis by a fibrocartilage. This joint is called the pubic symphysis.

The Fibrocartilage

The pubic symphysis has a flattened cylindrical, slightly oval shape. The two flattened surfaces join the side of each pubic bone, right and left, to the other.

The fibrocartilage is able to change shape just a bit.

The Ligaments of the Pubic Symphysis

In the front, back, top, and bottom of the fibrocartilage, ligaments run from one pubic bone to the other. They keep the two bones connected and prevent their separation.

These ligaments are very important during delivery, as they prevent excessive distension of the pubis.

When we talk about the pubis, it can have many meanings. Depending on the context, it can designate:

- An embryonic area of the iliac bone made up of the anterior third of the acetabulum and the bony parts situated in front of it
- The most anterior part of this bony region
- In the most current usage, the area where the two pubic bones join, or the pubic mound

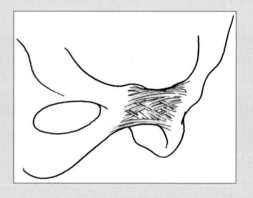

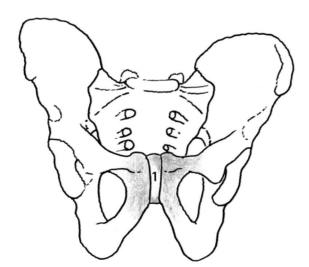

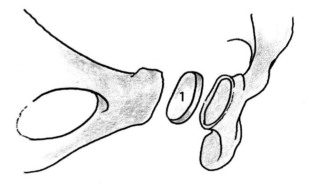

Here the joint is disassembled so we can see all of its different components.

How It's Imagined

The pubis is drawn as one solid block of bone without a joint or without fibrocartilage, and therefore without any apparent ability to move.

Sometimes the pubic bones are drawn without the fibrocartilage that joins them. The bones therefore have an open space between them.

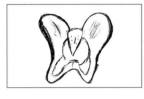
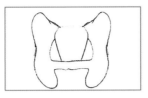
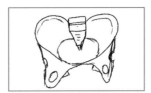

The pubis as one bone or missing the fibrocartilage

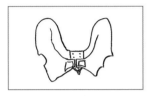
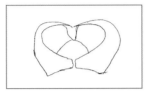
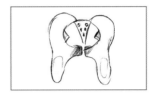

The pubis as two disjointed bones

The Pubic Symphysis Has a Special Role in Movement of the Pelvis

Because of its deformability, the fibrocartilage of the pubic symphysis has a mobility like that of the intervertebral disks (though a bit less)—like an accordion we might hold tightly between two hands.

Deformable in all directions, it is like a "rotation disk" that allows the iliac bones to move in all planes, echoing those of the sacroiliac joints and hips. *These are not large movements but multidirectional ones.*

On the day of delivery, the mobility of this joint is greatly augmented. How does the symphysis change shape during the passage of the fetus? Most often it is a combination of the enlarging of one area and the narrowing of another, for example:

- Squeezing at the bottom and opening at the top when the innominate lines move apart in the **(1)** engagement phase (see pp. 56 and 61)

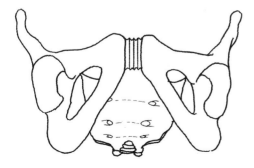

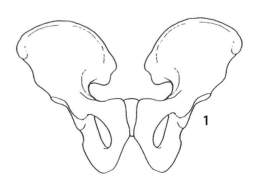

- Squeezing at the top and opening at the bottom with the opening of the outlet in the **(2)** final phase of expulsion (see pp. 57 and 62)

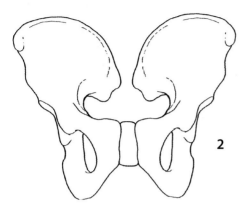

- Pinching or widening
- Twisting on itself in torsion, when the two iliac bones rotate in opposite directions in the **(3)** sagittal plane (such as when we walk)

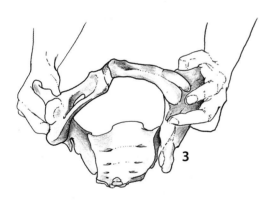

All of these movements can be combined. The fibrocartilage can be twisted, stretched, and pinched all at the same time, with asymmetrical changes in the shape of the pelvis (see p. 153).

see pp. 57 and 62; see p. 153

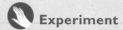

Experiment

You can feel these movements yourself by placing your hands on the symphysis while performing actions that mobilize the pelvis (for example, taking long strides when you walk).

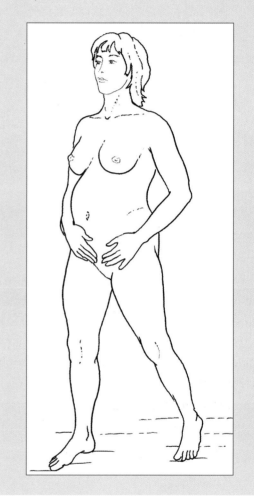

THE PELVIS ARTICULATES
WITH THE NEIGHBORING BONES

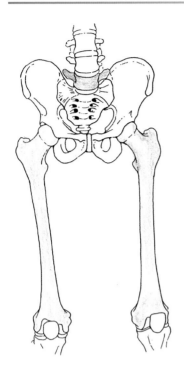

Changes in the pelvis are often caused by the actions of the neighboring bones.

- Each iliac bone works in close relationship with its corresponding femur.
- The sacrum moves in relation to the lower spinal vertebrae.

With the Spinal Column
(The Sacrolumbar Joint)

The sacrum is connected to the fifth lumbar vertebra, which is the lowest vertebra (L5). This forms the **sacrolumbar** joint or the **lumbosacral** joint (today we shorten it to L5/S1). The joint is actually made up of three different joints.

At the Front

The sacral plateau matches up with the inferior plateau of L5.

The junction of the sacrum and this vertebra is made by way of an **intervertebral disk,** the lowest on the spinal column. It has a special form: thinner in the back than in the front.

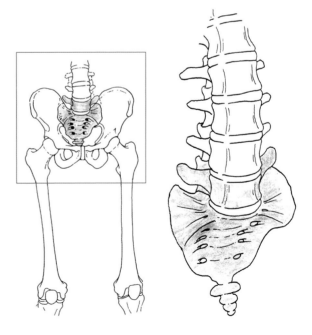

The vertebral body of L5 has somewhat the same form.

Because of the disk's ability to change shape, L5 can move on S1.

At the Back

At the back, on each side, are two small articulations called **(1)** interapophyseal joints. Each connects a small articular surface of the sacrum, which is circular, covered with cartilage, and directed backward, with a corresponding surface on the lower part of L5 that is rounded and directed forward. These two mini-joints are each held together by a small capsule and ligaments.

We find some important ligaments a bit removed from the sacrolumbar joint: these are the **(2)** iliolumbar ligaments that link the transverse processes of L4 and L5 to the iliac crest.

The superior ligament brakes contranutation (see p. 50), and the inferior ligament brakes nutation (see p. 46). These ligaments also restrict the lateral movement of the lower vertebral column.

During labor, the iliolumbar ligaments are put under pressure and are often the cause of pain at the top of the sacroiliac joints—a common complaint of many women.

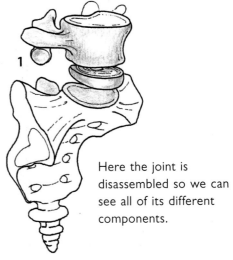

Here the joint is disassembled so we can see all of its different components.

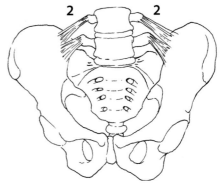

How It's Imagined

We are often surprised by the location of this hinge on our own body because many of us imagine that it is much higher. Here are three examples of drawings where this junction does not even appear.

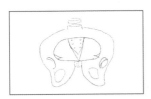 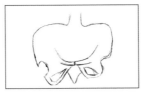 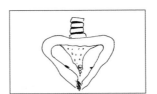

Confusion about the sacrolumbar junction

The Hip

The pelvis is connected to the lower limbs by the two **coxofemoral joints,** commonly known as the hips. These joints play an important role in the subject of this book. Our description of the hip covers only the aspects that are important for the mobility of the pelvis.

Two articulating surfaces come together in each hip.

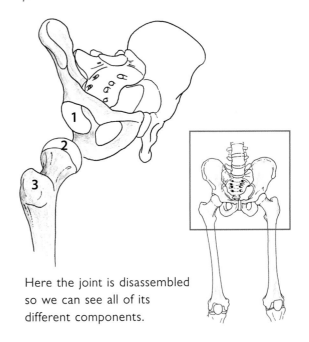

- On the iliac bone, the articulating surface takes the form of a cuplike hollow called the **cotyle** or the **(1)** acetabulum.
- At the upper end of the neck of the femur is the **(2)** femoral head, whose articulating surface is in the form of two-thirds of a sphere.

Here the joint is disassembled so we can see all of its different components.

The articulating surfaces are covered with thick cartilage. They are like a full sphere fitted into a hollow sphere.

The top of the femur is recognizable by a large protrusion, the **(3)** greater trochanter, on which we put weight when we lie on our side (see pp. 101 and 118).

The Location of the Hips

For the purposes of this book it is important to know that many people wrongly imagine that the hips are actually the top of the iliac crest at the waist.

Locate on Yourself

The simplest way to locate the coxofemoral joint is to trace a diagonal line from the ASIS to the pubis. A little before midway you arrive at the spot where the coxofemoral joint lies deep in the pelvis. Of course you cannot palpate the joint, because it is covered by the joint capsule, ligaments, and muscles, as well as vessels and nerves. It is from here that the pelvis can be mobilized in all directions.

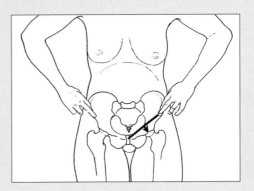

27

The Ligaments of the Hip Are Strong

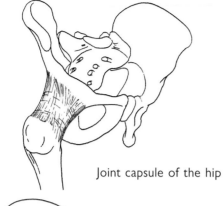

Joint capsule of the hip

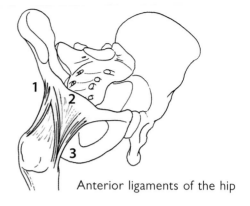

Anterior ligaments of the hip

- The **(1)** iliotrochanteric bundle
- The **(2)** iliopretrochantinian bundle
- The **(3)** pubofemoral bundle

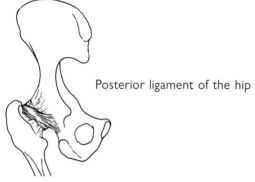

Posterior ligament of the hip

The hip joint is held securely within a fibrous sleeve that surrounds the femoral head and attaches to both the femoral neck and the rim of the acetabulum: this is the **joint capsule.**

The joint capsule is reinforced, especially in front, by three **ligaments** that are arranged in a zigzag pattern, in three bundles.

These ligaments are thick and strong. Because they attach to the pelvis, when they are tensed they cause the pelvis to move. These ligaments contribute to frequent changes in the shape of the pelvis, a fact that is very important to remember when considering the subject of this book (see p. 96).

The joint capsule is also reinforced by a posterior ligament, which, when under tension, moves the iliac bone (see p. 92).

How It's Imagined

When drawing the pelvis, people often omit the point where the pelvis articulates with the lower limbs. Often, too, when they try to locate the hip on their own body, they find themselves instead at the top of the iliac crest. They are surprised to realize that the hip is more anterior than they had imagined. Here are some examples of drawings that are missing the acetabulum.

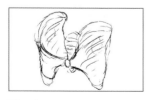 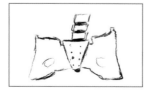 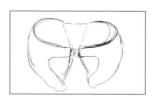

The hip joint: a big omission

The Pelvis Is Connected to the Trunk by Many Muscles

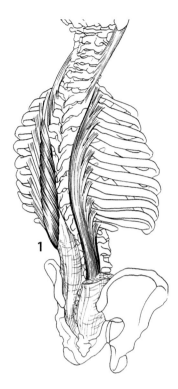

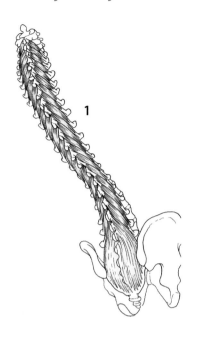

The muscles that attach the pelvis to the upper areas of the trunk* (principally to the spine and the thoracic rib cage) can all be found in the area around the waist. All of these muscles can pull on one or another of the pelvis's parts. The principal muscles are:

All the muscles here are cited for their action on the pelvis (see chapter 4).

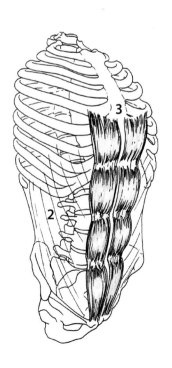

- The **(1)** back muscles, which can bring the sacrum into nutation (see p. 85) or the iliac bone into anteversion
- The **(2)** oblique abdominal muscles (designated here by lines), which can cause the iliac bone to incline
- The **(3)** rectus abdominus of the abdomen, which can pull the pubis into retroversion

---

*For a detailed description of these muscles, see the books *Anatomy of Movement* and *No- Risk Abs* by Blandine Calais-Germain (see the bibliography).

The Hip Is Covered by Numerous Muscles

The muscles of the hips connect the pelvis to the thighs. Together they form a dense muscular layer. During movement they, like the ligaments, become passive movers of the iliac bone. When contracted they can actively move the bone. To simplify the study of this area, we will look only at what we need to understand pelvic movement.

Flexion or Anteversion Muscles:

- **The psoas and iliacus** (not represented), which extend from the lumbar spine and the internal iliac fossa to the lesser trochanter*
- **The rectus femorus** (not represented), which runs from the anterior inferior iliac spine to the tibia
- **The gluteus minimus** (not represented), which runs from the external iliac fossa to the greater trochanter

Extension or Retroversion Muscles:

- The **(1)** gluteus maximus, which runs from the sacrum and the posterior gluteal line of the inner upper iliac bone to the back of the femur (on a crest called the linea aspera)
- The **(2)** hamstrings, which run from the ischium to the tibia and fibula
- The back part of the gluteus medius

3 Adductor Muscles:

- **(3)** Adductor muscles run from the ischio-pubic ramus to the femur (on the back of the femur on the linea aspera).

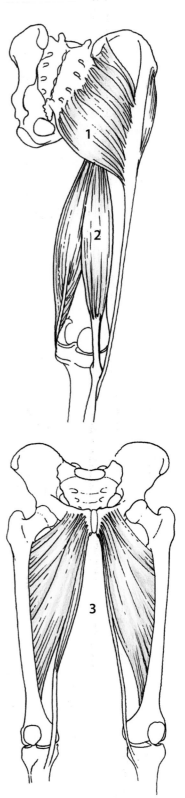

---

*The lesser projection is above and inside the femur.

30

Abductor Muscles:

- The **(4)** gluteus medius, which runs from the external iliac fossa to the greater trochanter of the femur
- The small muscles called the **(5)** deep external rotators, which cause external rotation

of the femur or internal rotation of the iliac bone (see p. 90)

All of these muscles can also participate in the **rotation** of the femur or the pelvis.

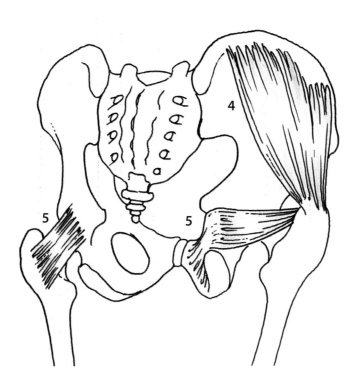

2
THE PARTS
OF THE PELVIS

Lesser Pelvis, Greater Pelvis

The internal pelvis is made of two parts, one stacked on the other. There is the *greater pelvis,* formed predominately by the wings of the iliac bone. It is large and open in the front. It holds the lower abdominal organs.

The *lesser pelvis* is formed by the sacrum and the lower half of the iliac bones. It is close to half the size of the greater pelvis, and more closed, and it contains the viscera of the lesser pelvis.

The Openings

In the lesser pelvis we can see three distinct zones that resemble irregular circles. These "circles" are called the *openings*—or inlets or outlets—depending on their position.

During pregnancy, the growing fetus stays in the greater pelvis. It crosses into the lesser pelvis during delivery.

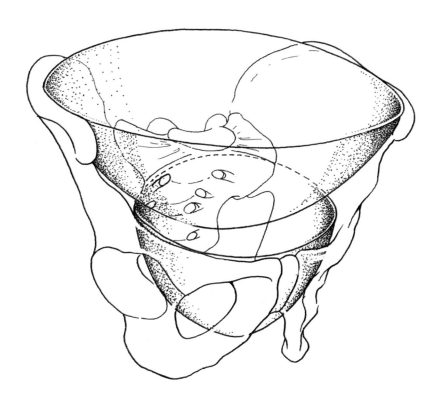

The Superior Opening

The superior opening marks the border between the greater pelvis and lesser pelvis. It is bounded by the anterior border of the sacral plateau, **the promontory of the sacrum,** and the anterior border of the **sacral wings,** which continue into the **iliopectineal lines** that terminate at the upper part of the pubis. The inlet takes the form of a circle or a heart shape. The span of this opening is important for the passage of the fetus.

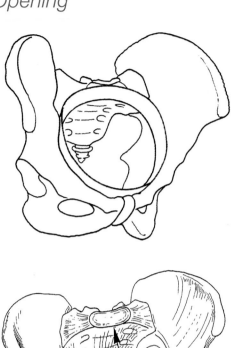

We measure the span of the superior opening in a pregnant woman with a manual exam that serves to determine the dimensions of the pelvis. This is sometimes followed up with an imaging procedure called pelvimetry. We specifically look at the **(1)** anteroposterior diameter, as well as two transverse dimensions.

- The **(2)** median transverse diameter
- The **(3)** effective diameter, a measurement taken behind the median transverse diameter

We will see in chapters 3 and 5 of this book how pelvic movements can change the anteroposterior diameter and, to a lesser extent, the transverse diameters.

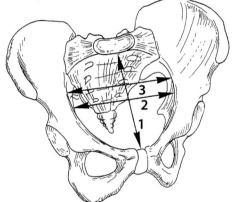

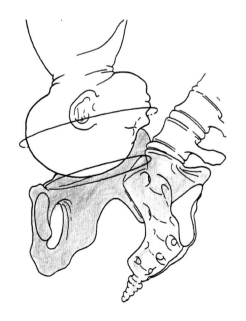

The Middle Opening

The middle opening is situated below the superior opening. It is delineated by the **back of the pubic symphysis,** the **ischial spines,** and **the front of the sacrum,** a bit above the level of the coccyx.

A determining factor in the shape and size of this opening is the size and direction of the ischial spines, which are sometimes more exaggerated in the way they protrude toward the interior (see p. 8).

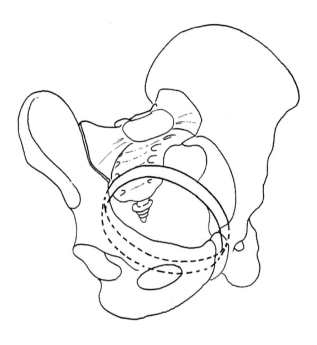
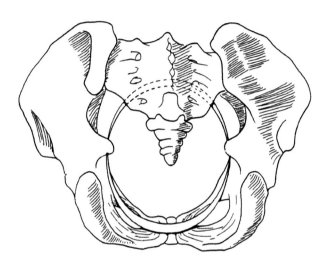

How It's Imagined

On page 4 we see a "butterfly" pelvis, flat and without volume.

Here, the pelvises are represented in three dimensions and with a certain sense of volume, but the interior is not clear: we see a single space, without the innominate line that signals the beginning of the lesser pelvis.

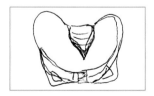
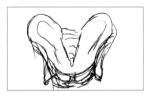
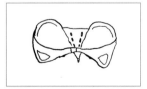

The openings: one enormous hole in the interior of the pelvis

The Inferior Opening

The inferior is the lowest opening, the last bony outlet that the fetus passes through before birth. It is formed by:

- The bottom of the pubic symphysis
- The ischio-pubic rami
- The two large sacrotuberous ligaments

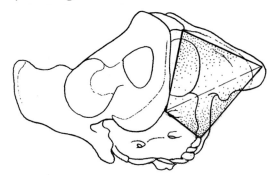

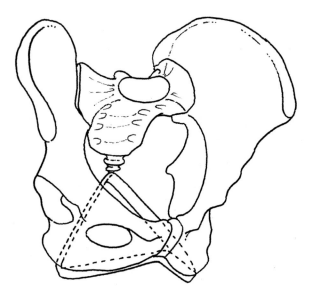

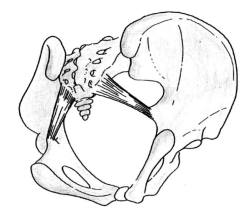

Taken as a whole, it is rhomboid in shape, or we can consider it as two triangles: one anterior urogenital triangle, oriented downward and toward the front; and a posterior anorectal triangle, oriented downward and toward the back.

The size and the shape of the **three pelvic openings can be modified by movement** of the pelvis. The inferior opening is the most modifiable. The middle opening can also change markedly. The superior opening is the least modifiable because it is located in the axis of movements of the sacroiliac. Nevertheless, it is transformable, especially asymmetrically.

How It's Imagined

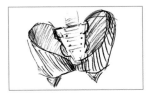

One imprecise opening

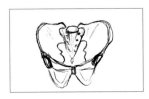

Four ischial spines instead of two

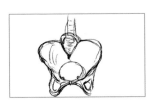

An opening below the coccyx

36

The Three Openings

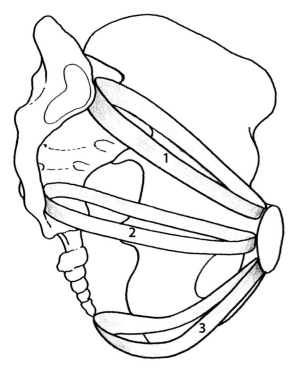

"After taking the 'Pelvis and Childbirth' work-shop, when we went back to work in the delivery room we looked at [each woman] in a different way, and we saw her pelvis in three dimensions. We visualized the movement of the fetus inside her pelvis. There's no going back. Nothing is as it was before."

CARMEN SANCHEZ
MIDWIFE, LORCA, MURCIE, SPAIN

"One woman, after her second delivery, said that what helped most with pushing the baby out was knowing the direction of the vagina between the ischio-pubic rami."

TERESA MARTINEZ, MIDWIFE, ALACANT HEALTH
CENTER, VALENCIA, SPAIN

With the pelvis in a vertical position, the three openings do not overlap but are arranged obliquely to each other: (1) the superior opening, (2) the middle opening, (3) and the inferior opening.

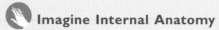

Sit on a chair with your feet flat on the floor and a bit separated. Feel the ischial tuberosities in contact with the seat. Place one hand at the pubic symphisis. Cup your other hand around the sacrum. The space that you perceive between your two hands corresponds to the totality of the pelvic cavity (see the definition on the next page).

Imagine a horizontal circle halfway up the pubis and the sacrum. The heat of your hands can help you sense where the borders of this circle are located. This circle designates the middle opening. When you are seated, it is horizontal.

Without losing your sense of the space between your hands, imagine another circle about the same size as the middle opening. It is at an oblique angle: it is higher in the back, at about the level of the heel of your hand (sacrolumbar level). In front, it meets the pubis, just a bit higher than the circle of the middle opening. This circle is the superior opening. This is the spot at which the fetus begins its passage to the outside world.

Finally, keeping your hands in contact with

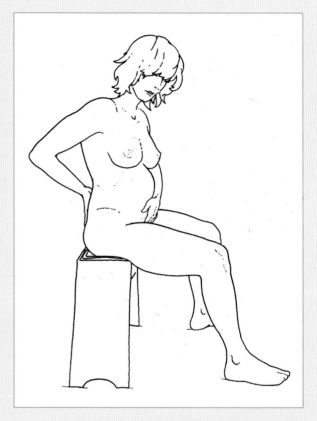

your pelvis, imagine a rhomboid with points at the bottom of the pubis, the two ischiums (which are pressing into the seat), and the coccyx (located at the tip of the middle finger of the hand that is cupping the sacrum). This is the inferior opening.

The Pelvic Cavity

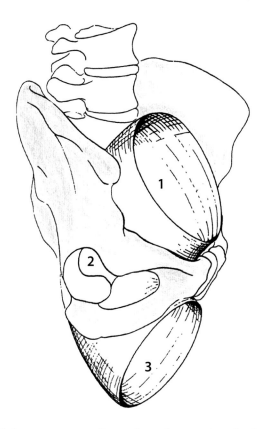

These openings form the pelvic cavity, the bony pathway in the lesser pelvis that the fetus must pass through.

This cavity takes the form of a **cylinder** passing through the openings. Because the openings are not parallel, the cylinder is **curved.**

Imagine Internal Anatomy

The Pelvic Cavity Is Like a Curved Pipe

You can use two images here:

- A curved pipe installed vertically
- A toy in the shape of a spring

In both images, which represent the path that the fetus takes, look for the entry, which corresponds to **(1)** the superior opening. The exit corresponds to the third circle, or **(3)** the inferior opening. Midway along the path is another circle that corresponds to **(2)** the middle opening.

By using these images, you can see that the three circles have a different orientation relative to one another, and as the fetus passes through them it takes not a straight path but a **curved one.** Now try to imagine these circles in your own pelvis.

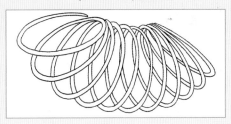

How It's Imagined

The channel of the pelvic cavity is often imagined and depicted as a straight pipe in the interior of the basin, even in obstetrics texts. Here are some drawings where the pelvic cavity is represented in this way.

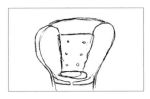 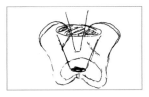 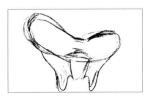

The pelvic cavity as a straight path

The Fetal Head "Turns" in the Lesser Pelvis

It Rotates at the Pubis

The fetus does not take a straight path but makes approximately a quarter turn.

- It enters through the superior opening, which runs obliquely upward and forward.
- It exits through the inferior opening, which runs obliquely downward and forward.
- Between the two openings, it turns at the pubis, following the concave curve of the sacrum in the back.

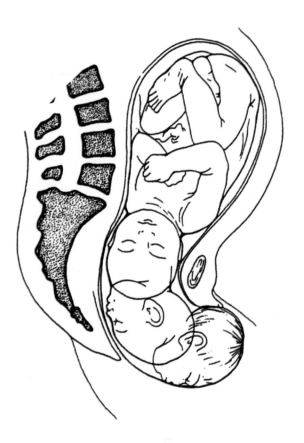

At the Same Time, It Turns Transversely

Why does it turn transversely? Because the diameter of the birth canal varies: the largest diameters of the openings are not oriented on the same plane.

The head of the fetus is not spherical but ovoid in form, and it "slips" through the pelvic cavity: at each step it must orient its shortest diameter in the longest diameter of each opening, and at the end it turns on itself.

In the most favorable circumstances:

- To pass through the superior opening, wider than it is long, the head turns to the side (usually to the right, though it can turn to the left).
- To pass through the middle opening, longer than it is wide, the head turns to the front, with the fetus's face turned toward the mother's sacrum.

The mother's pelvis can accompany and facilitate the rotations of the fetal head, or at least not thwart it.

Helpful Terms

Asynclitism

When the fetal head engages in the superior opening, the term *asynclitism* describes a situation where the sagittal suture of the head (momentarily placed in the frontal plane by the head's rotation) is not equidistant from the pubis and the sacrum but instead moves closer to one or the other.

Disengagement

Disengagment marks the phase when the fetal head emerges from the inferior opening.

Dystocia, eutocia

The word *dystocia* references the problems and difficulties that can arise in the course of the progression of the fetus through the birth canal. It is the opposite of the word *eutocia,* which means a spontaneous delivery that ends with the spontaneous expulsion of a fetus that has not suffered any detrimental effects.

Engagement

Engagement marks the phase when the fetal head crosses the superior opening.

Ligament

A ligament is a fibrous tissue that connects two bones at a joint. Most often, it is a thickening of the joint capsule. The ligament is rich in collagen fibers and resistant to traction. It also contains many nerve endings that are sensitive to tension, pressure, and pain. The excessive compression and stretching of ligaments during childbirth triggers pain.

Pronation, supination of the iliac bones

In this book, *pronation* and *supination* designate the movement of the iliac bones in the frontal-transverse plane. We illustrate these internal movements by comparing them to the movements of the hands in reference to the forearms (see pp. 60–62).

Slip

In this book, *slip* refers to the movement of the fetus as it passes between the bones of the birth canal. This passage can be assisted by alternating the movements of the bones.

Unrestricted pelvis

We're speaking here about the pelvis being free to move around the heads of the femurs, that is to say, at the hip joints.

When we speak of the unrestricted pelvis, we are considering the entire pelvis with its four bones stable in relationship to one another. We consider that the pelvis is moving like a solid piece. When the pelvis is put in motion it can move in three orthogonal planes (frontal, sagittal, and transverse) and in all the intermediate planes (see pp. 43 and 147). At the same time the two iliac bones, being free, can change position when they are pushed on by the head of the fetus.

3

HOW DOES
THE PELVIS MOVE?

The Intrinsic Movements

Describing Movements of the Pelvis

The Three Orthogonal* Planes

The movements of the pelvis, as well as the rest of the body, can be studied from three points of view that allow us to observe motion possibilities in **three planes.**

- **The sagittal plane** covers movements visible *in profile* that go toward the front or back, for example, flexion of the hip or of the spine.
- **The frontal plane** covers movements visible *from the front* that are made away from or toward the midline of the body, for example, abduction (raising) or adduction (lowering) of the leg to the side.
- **The transverse plane** covers movements visible *from above or below* a person who is standing or lying, for example, internal or external rotation of the hips.

The Anatomical Reference Position

All of the movements described over the course of this chapter are begun in a standing position with the feet together and pointing forward.

The Movements Are Described as Symmetrical

In childbirth the pelvis often changes its form asymmetrically for several reasons.

- One of the sacroiliac joints or hips is more mobile than the other.
- The forces that cause pelvic movements (see chapter 5) are asymmetrical (for the simple fact, for example, that a laboring mother is right- or left-handed).
- The fetal head "passes" asymmetrically.

Still, to understand these movements, we need a point of reference, and it is simpler to consider the movements as symmetrical. We also need to imagine that:

- If the sacrum is mobile, the iliac bones are fixed.
- If the iliac bones are mobile, with identical mobility on both the right and left sides, the sacrum is fixed.

It is never really like this in practice. The following pages are intended simply to clarify the movements, which most often occur in combination with one another and asymmetrically.

The Four Planes of Hodge

In this book we will make reference to the steps that mark the passage of the fetal head through the pelvis. These steps correspond to the four planes cited by Hodge that are used in obstetrics.

> The orthogonal planes, practical for this study, do not correspond to normal movements, especially during childbirth. Most often they are cited in combination.

> Standing with your feet together and pointing forward is not a natural position, but this is the conventional starting position used in anatomy to describe movement.

---

*The orthogonal planes are at right angles to each other.

Intrinsic and Extrinsic Movements

When the pelvis moves in itself, articulating between its own bones, this is called an **intrinsic movement.**

When the pelvis moves in relation to its neighbors, this is called an **extrinsic movement.**

Only intrinsic movements directly modify the form of the pelvic cavity. Extrinsic movements, when they reach a certain level, can cause intrinsic movements. But this causality does not necessarily happen and not in a direct way.

Intrinsic movements of the pelvis are minimal in daily life. They occur most often at the same time as movements of the pelvis on the femur heads and movements of the lumbar spine, because these areas are connected anatomically. Because of this connection these intrinsic movements can be confused with extrinsic movements.

Because our study is focused on the pelvis, this chapter will detail how to distinguish between these two types of movements.

In this chapter we observe only the sequence of pelvic movements, without questioning what may cause them, which is discussed in chapter 5. Here we will look at specific circumstances that may, during delivery, inhibit the described movements.

> Intrinsic movements are not common and are only seen in childbirth or where there is exceptional mobility between the bones. They are not observed in a postural context where the pelvis is stable in a stance position or in osteopathic micro-movements of the pelvis.

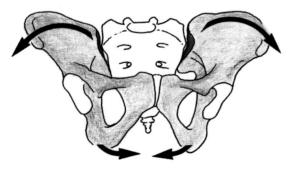

Abduction of the iliac is an example of intrinsic movement (see p. 56).

(see p. 56)

> Intrinsic movements can be caused by movement of the extrinsic joints. But to avoid confusion, we will look at this a second time.

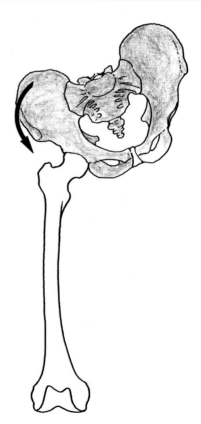

External lateral inclination of the pelvis is an example of extrinsic movement.

INTRINSIC MOVEMENTS OF THE PELVIS
IN THE SAGITTAL PLANE

Recall that movements in the sagittal plane are those that can be viewed in profile. These are the easiest to understand.

For the pelvis, the movements of the sacrum in the sagittal plane are those that are the best known and most often described.

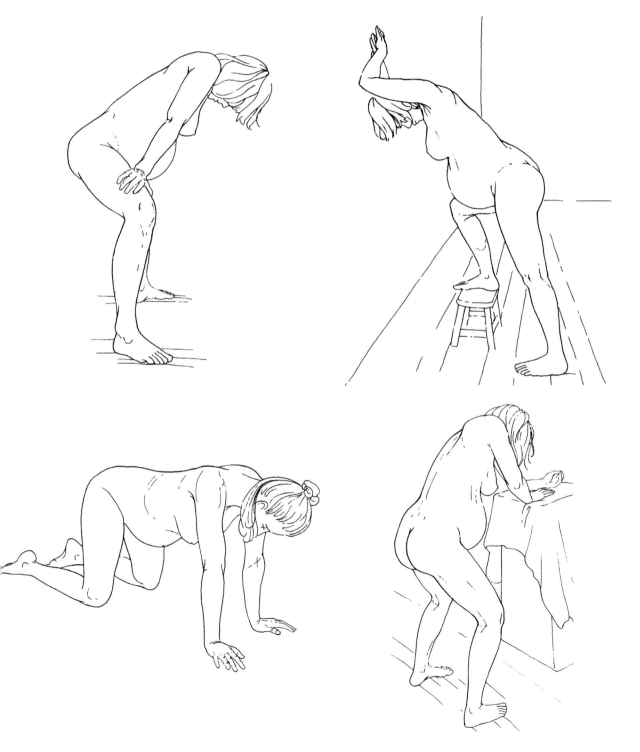

Nutation of the Sacrum or Sacral Nutation

Sacral nutation, as described in obstetrics texts, refers to displacement of the sacrum, specifically in the context of childbirth.

In sacral nutation the top of the sacrum tilts *forward*. The sacral promontory moves *closer* to the pubis and *descends* slightly. Conversely, the tailbone moves *away* from the pubic bone and slightly *upward*.

This movement happens primarily in the sacroiliac joints. It increases the distance between the coccyx and the pubis.

Sacral nutation is of importance during the expulsion phase, the period of disengagement (passage through the third and fourth planes), because it enlarges the inferior opening.

Support of the maternal pelvis at the lower part of the sacrum can inhibit this movement. It is therefore important during the disengagement phase to avoid pressure on the coccyx and the lower half of the sacrum, whether in a supine position (the end of the delivery table needs to be released) or in a seated position (there should not be pressure from behind on the lower half of the sacrum).*

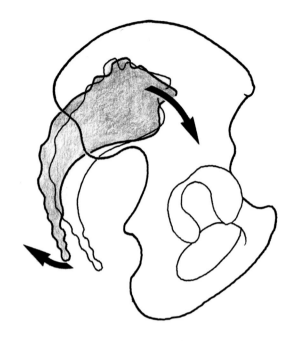

The word *nutation* designates either the movement described here or the normal position of the sacrum between the iliac bones, a little tipped to the front.

---

*This is particularly important if the final stage of the delivery takes place on a birthing chair.

Sacral Nutation

The amplitude of the movements is exaggerated for clarity.

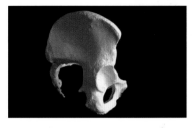 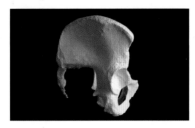 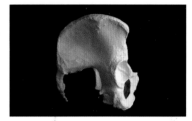

Viewed in profile (pelvis vertical). The sacrum tilts, promontory forward, coccyx backward.

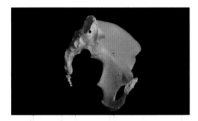 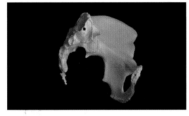 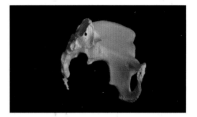

Viewed in profile, the right iliac removed. The sacrum tilts, promontory forward, coccyx backward.

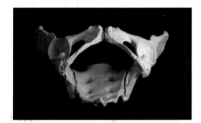 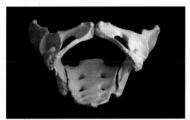 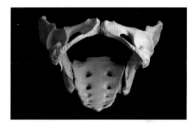

Inferior view (as if the woman is lying on her back). We see the coccyx move away from the pubis.

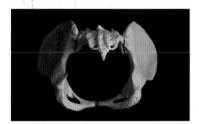 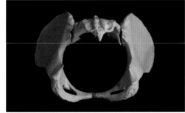 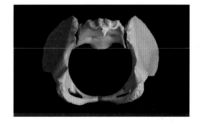

Inferior view (as if the woman is on all fours). The inferior opening enlarges sagittally.

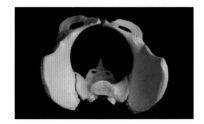 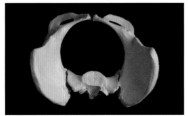 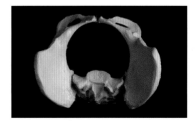

Superior view (from above). We see the promontory move closer to the pubis. The superior opening narrows sagittally.

Nutation of the Iliac or Iliac Nutation

Movements of the sacrum transform the pelvic cavity. But the same changes can be caused by the movement of the iliac bones around the sacrum.

To simplify, imagine that the two iliac bones move symmetrically and the sacrum remains stationary.

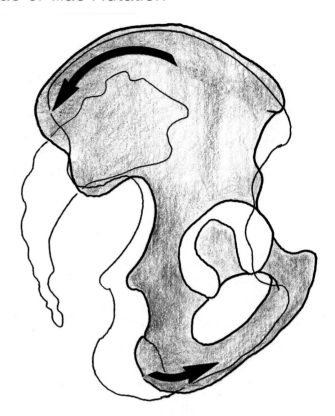

In this movement the iliac bones pivot around the sacrum. The ASIS tips *backward,* and the ischium tips *forward.* As with sacral nutation, the pubis moves *closer* to the sacral plateau, and conversely, the pubis moves *away* from the coccyx.

Here, too, the movement takes place principally in the sacroiliac. Here, too, we can see that it increases the distance between the coccyx and the pubis. Nutation of the iliac bones is a vital movement at the end of the expulsion phase, during disengagement, because it enlarges the inferior opening.

It is also an important movement (although to a lesser degree) in the passage of the fetus through the middle opening (second and third planes): if the ischial spines inhibit the passage of the fetus, nutation of the iliac can move one or both out of the way.

We'll see specifically on pages 94, 116, 140, and 141 how this movement is most often caused or enabled by traction coming from the femurs.

Iliac nutation, which happens in the sacroiliac between the bones of the pelvis, must not be confused with pelvic retroversion, which is a movement in the same direction but is produced at the hip joint. Retroversion of the pelvis does not change the form of the pelvis or the pelvic cavity.

Iliac Nutation

The amplitude of the movements is exaggerated for clarity.

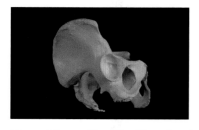 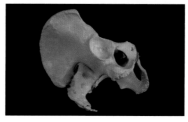 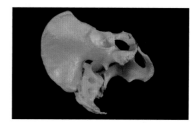

Viewed in profile. The iliac tilts, ischium forward, ASIS backward.

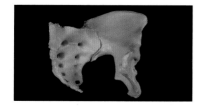 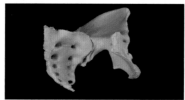 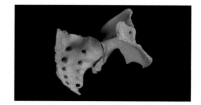

Viewed in profile, the right iliac removed. The left iliac tilts, ischium forward, ASIS backward.

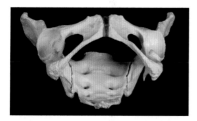 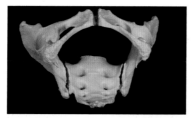 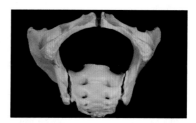

Inferior view (as if the woman is lying on her back). We see the pubis move away from the coccyx.

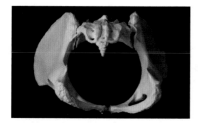 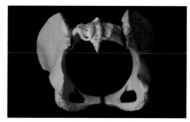 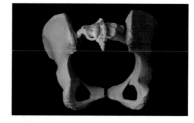

Inferior view (as if the woman is on all fours). The inferior opening enlarges sagittally.

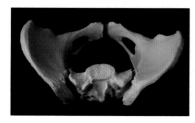 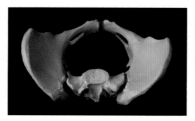 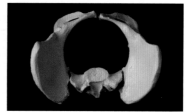

Superior view (from above). We see the promontory move closer to the pubis. The superior opening narrows sagittally (less visible here because the iliac is viewed at an oblique angle).

49

Contranutation of the Sacrum
or Sacral Contranutation

In sacral contranutation, the sacrum tilts to the *back*. The sacral plateau and the promontory move *away* from the pubis and *lift* slightly. Conversely, the coccyx moves *closer* to the pubis and *drops* slightly.

> Sacral contranutation, as described in obstetrics texts, refers to displacement of the sacrum, specifically in the context of childbirth.

This movement is made principally at the level of the sacroiliac. It increases the distance between the sacral promontory and the pubis.

Sacral contranutation is an interesting movement during the start of dilation, in the engagement phase (first plane), because it enlarges the superior opening sagittally, allowing the fetus to slip into the passage.

We'll see specifically on pages 85, 98, and 105 how sacral contranutation can be caused or enabled.

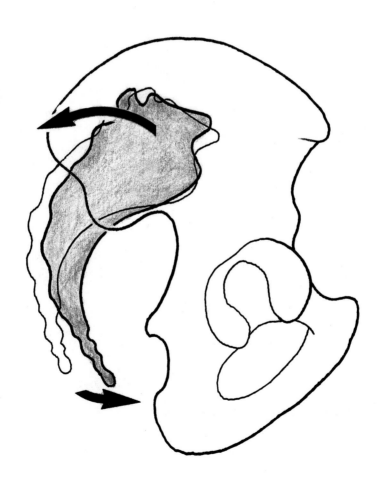

Sacral Contranutation

The amplitude of the movements is exaggerated for clarity.

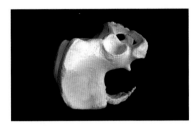 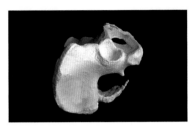 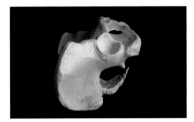

Viewed in profile. The sacrum tilts, promontory backward, coccyx forward.

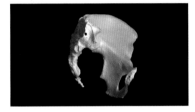 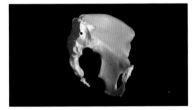 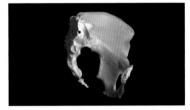

Viewed in profile, the right iliac removed. The sacrum tilts, promontory backward, coccyx forward.

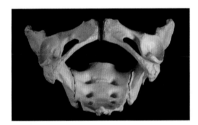 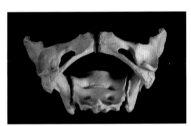 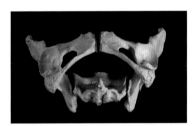

Inferior view (as if the woman is lying on her back). We see the coccyx move closer to the pubis.

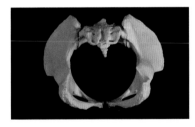 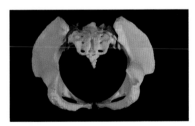 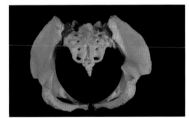

Inferior view (as if the woman is on all fours). The inferior opening narrows sagittally.

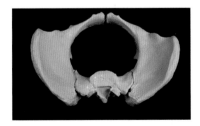 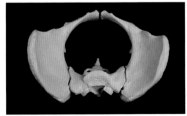 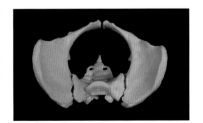

Superior view (from above). We see the promontory move away from the pubis. The superior opening enlarges sagittally.

51

Contranutation of the Iliac or Iliac Contranutation

To simplify, imagine that the two iliac bones move symmetrically and the sacrum remains stationary.

Here, too, the changes in shape caused by the movement of the sacrum can also be caused by the movement of the iliac bones around the sacrum.

In this movement, the iliac bones pivot around the sacrum. The ASIS tips *forward,* and the ischium tips *backward.*

As in sacral contranutation, the pubis moves *away* from the sacral plateau and promontory and *closer* to the coccyx.

Here, too, the movement takes place primarily in the sacroiliac joints. Here, too, we observe that it increases the distance between the promontory and the pubis; that is to say, it increases the sagittal diameter of the superior opening.

Contranutation of the iliac bones is a pertinent movement at the beginning of the dilation phase, at the time of engagement (passage through the first plane), because it enlarges the superior opening from front to back and allows the fetal head to position itself at the opening of the pelvic cavity.

We will see specifically on page 96 how this iliac contranutation can be caused or enabled.

Iliac contranutation, which happens in the sacroiliac between the bones of the pelvis, must not be confused with pelvic anteversion, which is a movement in the same direction but is produced at the hip joint. Anteversion of the pelvis does not change the form of the pelvis or the pelvic cavity.

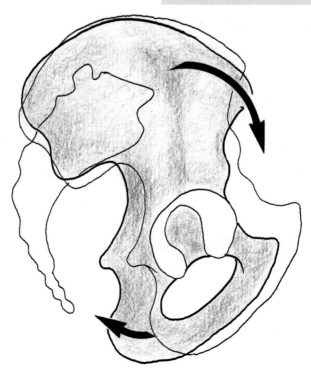

Iliac Contranutation

The amplitude of the movements is exaggerated for clarity.

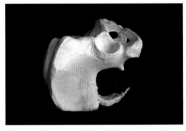 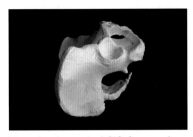 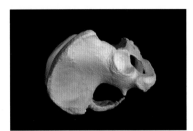

Viewed in profile. The iliac tilts, ischium backward, ASIS forward.

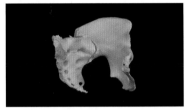 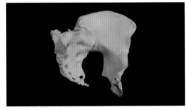 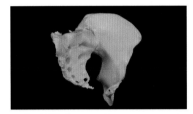

Viewed in profile, the right iliac removed. The iliac tilts, ischium backward, ASIS forward.

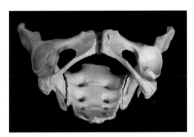 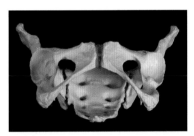 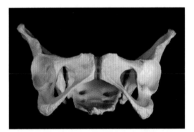

Inferior view (as if the woman is lying on her back). We see the pubis move closer to the coccyx.

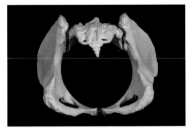 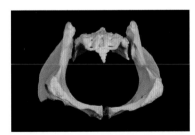 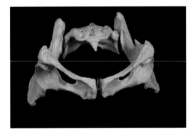

Inferior view (as if the woman is on all fours). The inferior opening narrows sagittally.

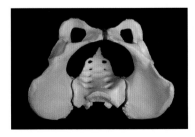 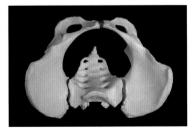 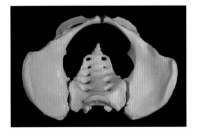

Superior view (from above). We see the pubis move away from the promontory. The superior opening enlarges sagittally.

INTRINSIC MOVEMENTS OF THE PELVIS
IN THE FRONTAL AND TRANSVERSE PLANES

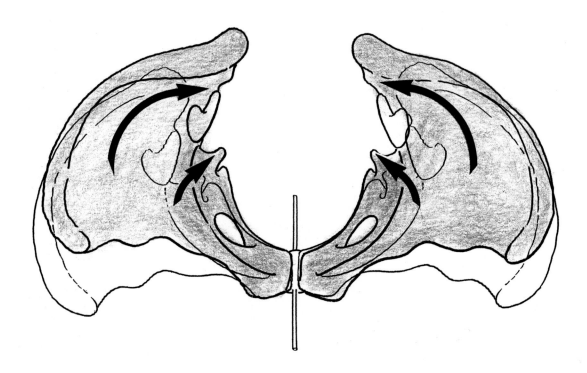

The following four pages help us understand, in detail, frontal and transverse movements. Those who do not want to go into
this much detail can turn directly to page
60, "Combined Movements in the Frontal-
Transverse Plane."

In the pages that follow we will look at movements made by the iliac bones that are much
less well known. These movements are important during childbirth because they transform
the pelvic cavity, although in a very different
way from those movements already discussed.

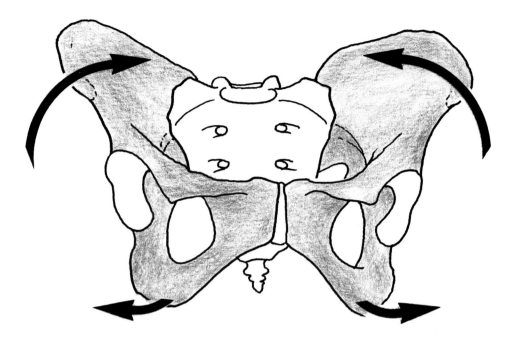

For all intents and purposes, the movements of the iliac bones appear to be very similar. When we learn precisely how to tell the difference among them, we can see that the effect is not the same, and sometimes opposite in a detail.

To simplify, we will imagine that the two iliac bones move symmetrically and the sacrum remains stationary.

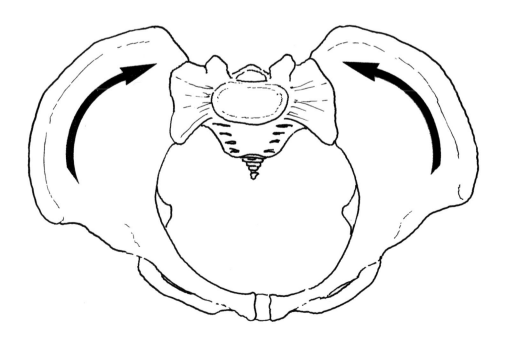

Movements in the Frontal Plane
(Abduction of the Iliac)

This movement is not described in obstetrics texts. The term *abduction of the iliac,* or *iliac abduction,* is part of the vocabulary original to the methods of the authors of this book.

Abduction of the iliac bones is a vital movement at the start of the engagement phase (first plane), because it pushes the innominate lines farther apart and enlarges the frontal diameter (called the transverse diameter) of the superior opening.

We'll see how the movement is caused or encouraged by traction coming from the femurs (p. 88) or from pressure (p. 100).

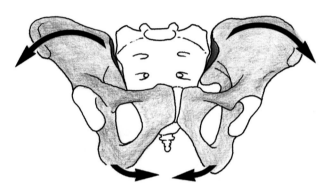

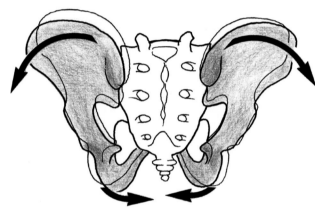

In iliac abduction the iliac bones pivot around the sacrum. The ASIS tilts *laterally,* to the outside, and the ischium tilts *medially,* to the inside.

The movement occurs simultaneously in

- The sacroiliac joints, which open at the top and close at the bottom
- The pubic symphysis, which widens at the top and narrows at the bottom

These two pages are for those who want to understand the intrinsic frontal movements of the pelvis in detail. Those who do not want to go into such great detail can turn directly to page 58.

Movements in the Frontal Plane
(Adduction of the Iliac)

This movement is not described in obstetrics text. The term *adduction of the iliac*, or *iliac adduction*, is part of the vocabulary original to the methods of the authors of this book.

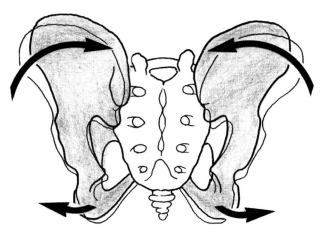

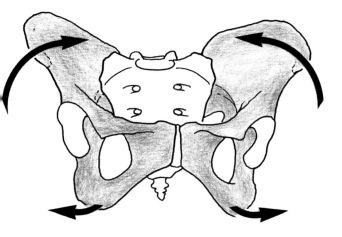

In iliac adduction the iliac bones pivot around the sacrum. The ASIS tips inward, *medially*, and the ischium tips outward, *laterally.*

The movement occurs simultaneously in

- The sacroiliac joints, which close at the top and open at the bottom
- The pubic symphysis, which narrows at the top and widens at the bottom

Adduction of the iliac bones is a vital movement at the end of expulsion—in the disengagement phase—because it separates the two ischia and enlarges the pelvic outlet.

To a lesser degree it is an important movement as the fetus passes the third plane, because it widens the ischial spines, however minimally.

We'll see how the movement is caused or encouraged by traction coming from the femurs (p. 86) or from external pressure on the iliac crest (p. 105).

Movements in the Transverse Plane
(Internal Rotation of the Iliac)

These two pages (58–59) are for those who want to understand the intrinsic transverse movements of the pelvis in great detail. Those who do not want to go into such detail can turn directly to page 58.

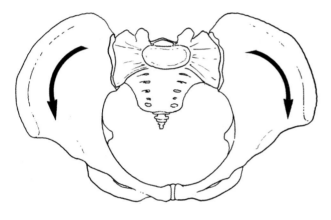

In internal iliac rotation the iliac bones pivot around a vertical axis that passes through the pubis. The ASIS moves *medially* and the PSIS moves *laterally*.

The movement occurs simultaneously in

- The sacroiliac joints, which spread, especially in the back
- The pubic symphysis, which narrows

The internal rotation of the iliac bones is an important movement for passage through the middle opening (third and fourth planes), because it opens the ischial spines and causes them to turn outward.

This movement is also important during the engagement phase (passage through the first plane), because it widens the space in the back, between the iliac bones, which encourages the sacrum to go into contranutation.

We'll see specifically on page 90 how the movement is caused or encouraged by traction coming from the femurs (the thighs).

This movement is not described in obstetrics texts. The term *internal rotation of the iliac bones* is part of the vocabulary original to the methods of the authors of this book.

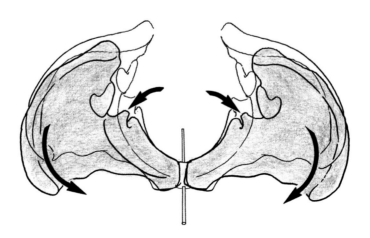

Movements in the Transverse Plane
(External Rotation of the Iliac)

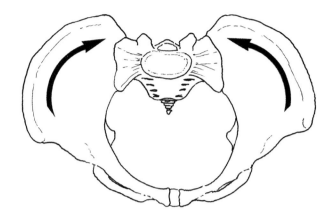

In external iliac rotation the iliac bones pivot around a vertical axis passing through the pubis. The ASIS moves *outward* and the PSIS moves *inward*.

The movement occurs simultaneously in

- The sacroiliac joints, which move closer to each other
- The pubic symphysis, which distends

The external rotation of the iliac is sometimes an important movement for passage through the middle opening (second and third planes), if it is alternated with internal rotation (which causes the ischial spines to move closer together and turn medially). The goal is to move the ischial spines in one direction and then the other, asymmetrically, which can encourage the passage of the fetal head.

We'll see specifically on page 91 how this movement can be caused or encouraged by traction coming from the femurs (the thighs).

This movement is not described in obstetrics texts. The term *external rotation of the iliac bones* is part of the vocabulary original to the methods of the authors of this book.

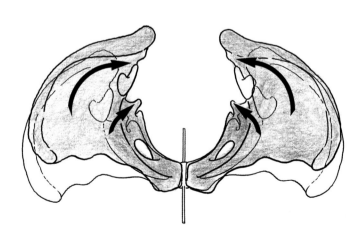

INTRINSIC MOVEMENTS OF THE
PELVIS IN THE FRONTAL-TRANSVERSE PLANE

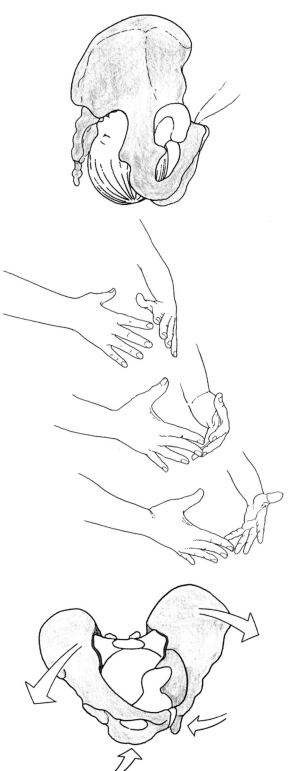

The movements that we have looked at do not occur often in just one orthogonal plane—strictly in the frontal plane, for example, or strictly in the transverse plane. Most often they occur in a combination of the two. In this book these movements are also called **pronation** and **supination,** in reference to the movements the hands can make around the axis of the forearms.

For the iliac bones, the movements of pronation and supination are made around an oblique axis that passes through the endpoints of the innominate line.

- The upper end of the sacroiliac joint in the back
- The top of the pubic symphysis in the front

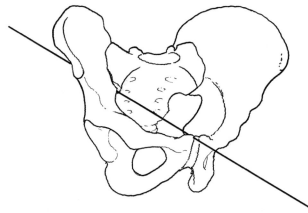

Supination of the Iliac

In supination the iliac bones pivot around an oblique axis that passes through the innominate line. The ASIS moves *outward* and a bit *forward,* and the ischium moves *inward* and a bit *backward.*

The movement occurs simultaneously in

- The sacroiliac joints, which open, especially at the top
- The pubic symphysis, which widens at the top and narrows at the bottom

Supination of the iliac bones is an important movement for passage through the superior opening (first plane), because it pushes the innominate lines farther apart. When alternated asymmetrically with pronation, supination facilitates the descent of the fetus through the middle opening and the inferior opening (second and third planes) and allows it to slip through (see pp. 114, 120–21, 123, and 133). This is especially important if the laboring mother has had an epidural.

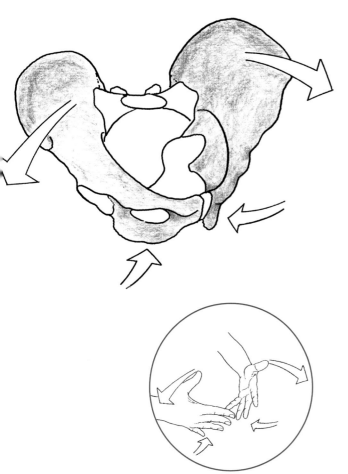

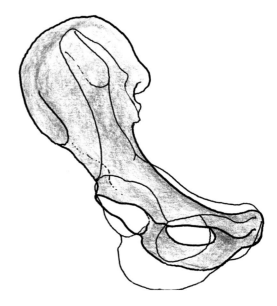

We'll see specifically on pages 93 and 141 how this movement can be encouraged principally by traction coming from flexion and external rotation of the femurs (the thighs).

Pronation of the Iliac

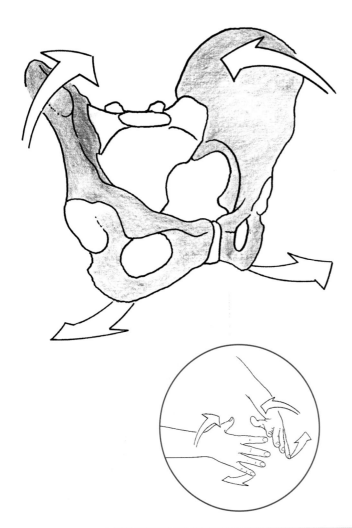

In pronation the iliac bones pivot around an oblique axis that passes though the ends of the innominate lines. The ASIS moves *inward* and a bit *backward,* and the ischium moves *outward* and a bit *forward.*

The movement occurs simultaneously in

- The sacroiliac joints, which open, especially at the bottom
- The pubic symphysis, which narrows at the top and widens at the bottom

Pronation of the iliac bones is an important movement for passage through the middle opening and the inferior opening (third and fourth planes), because it separates the ischial spines frontally and transversally at the same time.

We'll see specifically on pages 92 and 116 how this movement can be caused or encouraged essentially by traction coming from flexion and internal rotation of the femurs (the thighs).

These two movements, pronation and supination of the iliac, are not described in obstetrics texts. The terms *iliac pronation* and *iliac supination* are part of the vocabulary original to the methods of the authors of this book.

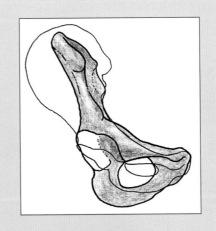

The Four Stages of Childbirth
and the Movements of the Pelvis

Before the First Step

The head is free and the fetus still above the superior opening. What does the pelvis do?

The pelvis gets ready and opens "at the top."

In practical terms, if the woman is resting, she can achieve contranutation by

• Relaxing the back muscles
• Keeping pressure off the top of the sacrum

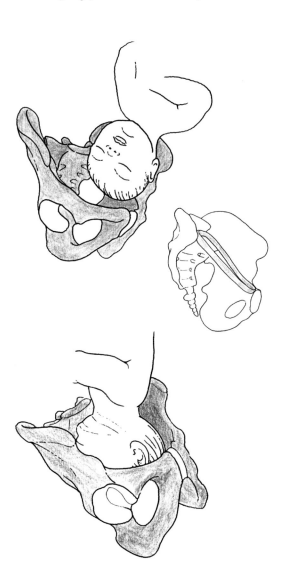

It is desirable for the woman to find a position where gravity is going to help (vertical).

In practical terms, if the woman is moving, she can choose free pelvic movements starting from the three "star positions" (see chapter 8) and small tilting and transition movements (see chapter 7).

First Step

The fetus crosses the superior opening. What does the pelvis do?

The superior opening has to enlarge by

• Sacral or iliac contranutation
• Opening of the innominate lines to enlarge the superior opening laterally (iliac abduction and/or iliac supination)

In practical terms, if the woman is resting, we can encourage contranutation by

• Relaxing the back muscles
• Keeping pressure off the upper part of the sacrum
• Applying heat to and around the sacrum

It is desirable for the woman to change positions when necessary.

In practical terms, if the woman is moving, she can choose free pelvic movements starting from the "star positions" (see chapter 8), specifically transition movements (see chapter 7).

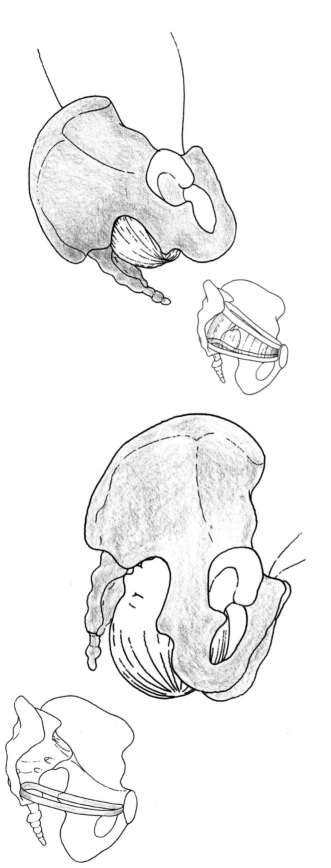

Second Step

The fetus crosses the zone between the superior opening and the ischial spines. What does the pelvis do?

The middle opening needs to enlarge at the back and laterally: the ischial spines have to open and turn outward (nutation, and at the same time internal rotation or pronation of the iliac bones).

In practical terms, if the woman is resting, she should avoid lying on her back in favor of

- Lying on her side
- Being on all fours

She should use external rotation and internal rotation of the femurs, alternating the asymmetries, rocking, and transition of the pelvis (see chapter 7) to move the ischial spines.

In practical terms, if the woman is moving, she can choose movements in the three "star positions" (see chapter 8), using external rotation and internal rotation of the femurs, alternating the asymmetries to move the ischial spines.

In this book, we make reference to the steps of the passage of the fetal head through the pelvis. These steps correspond to the four planes of Hodges referred to in obstetrics.

Third Step

The fetus passes the ischial spines. What does the pelvis do?

The middle opening needs to enlarge in the front and in the back.

In practical terms, if the woman is resting, she can encourage the opening of the lower pelvis by:

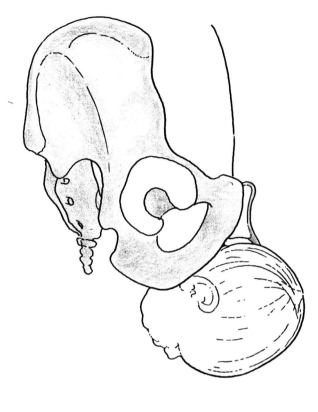

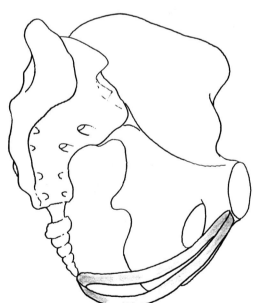

- Lying on her side
- Being on all fours, with flexion and internal rotation of the femurs

In practical terms, if the woman if moving, she can choose movements from the three "star positions" (see chapter 8), emphasizing internal rotation of the femurs, and alternating asymmetries to open the ischial spines and the ischial tuberosities.

Fourth Step

The fetus passes the pelvic outlet. This is the final step. What does the pelvis do?

The inferior opening needs to widen between the ischia, while at the same time maintaining its opening sagittally.

In practical terms, no pressure should be put on the lower part of the sacrum. The woman can adopt a position where one or both femurs are in a large degree of flexion, while also employing abduction and internal rotation, or even a vertical position, with or without suspending herself from a support, where the "free pelvis" will change its interior shape.

4

HOW DOES THE AREA AROUND THE PELVIS MOVE?

The Extrinsic Movements

This chapter looks at how the pelvis moves in relation to the neighboring structures.

- The spine above
- The femurs below

The Pelvis Moves with the Spine

Between the sacrum and the lumbar vertebra L5, movements are principally to the *back:* the vertebra L5 can move in extension at the sacral plateau, or the sacrum can tilt to the back when the coccyx is lifted (this looks like nutation).

The inverse movement (tilting L5 forward, or tilting the sacrum and coccyx forward) is more limited because the form of the intervertebral disk, being higher in the front than in the back, does not favor this movement.

Lateral movements are almost nonexistent, because they are restricted by the iliolumbar ligaments. *Rotation,* too, is almost nonexistent, restricted by the bony limits of the joint.

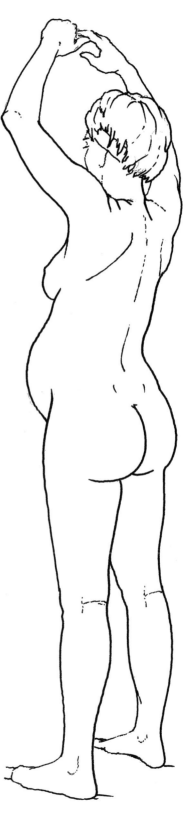

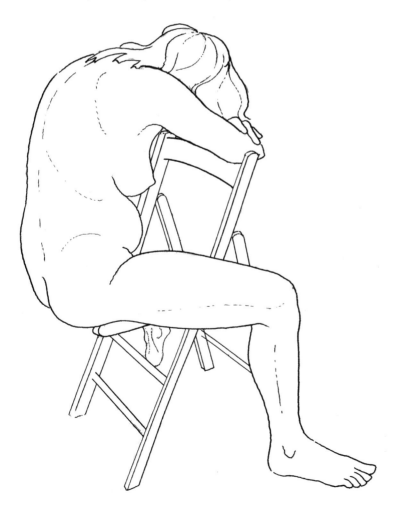

At the Hip

The Femur Can Move in All Directions*

The surfaces of the hip joint are like a full sphere encased in a hollowed-out sphere. This form allows the femur to move in all directions.

On the day of delivery we often ask a laboring mother for unusual movements of the femur, movements that she would otherwise rarely make, or we ask for greater amplitude of a movement than usual.

The Iliac Bone Can Move in All Directions*

However—and this is very important to the topic of this book—all of the movements that the femur is capable of can be made by the iliac bone (or by the pelvis, if the two iliac bones move simultaneously). It can move in all directions on the femoral head. Iliac movement is of major importance in changing the form of the pelvic cavity. And this is why, in the following pages, hip movements will be presented first as "made by the pelvis."

To adjust the form of the pelvis at the time of delivery, the most interesting positions are those that allow for mobility of the iliac bone. We call these "unrestricted" pelvic positions (see p. 41):

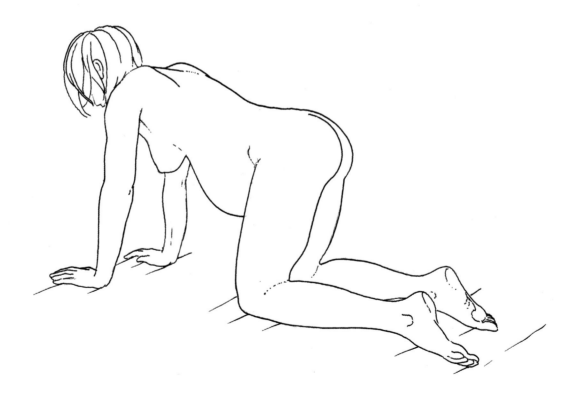

---

*As long as the joint does not meet with ligament or muscle tension.

- Lying on the side (see pp. 118–24)
- On the knees and all variations (see p. 129)
- Standing with knees slightly bent (see p. 135)
- Sitting on a ball (see p. 128)

We will find these positions again in the pages devoted to the three "star positions" (see chapter 8).

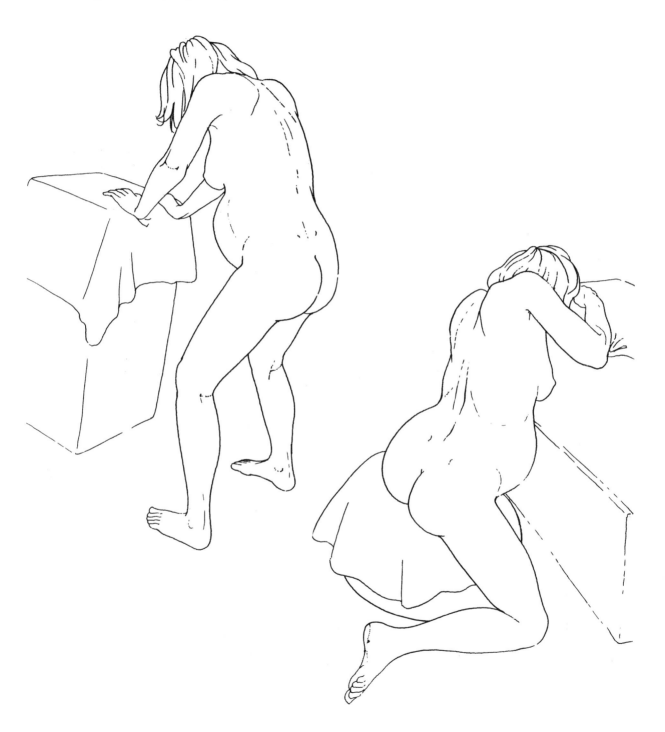

Movement of the Pelvis to the Back or Front
(Anteversion and Retroversion)

Anteversion is a movement of the entire pelvis at the hips. The reference point is the ASIS, which moves *lower* and *forward,* while at the same time the ischium moves *backward.*

Retroversion is also a movement of the entire pelvis at the hips. The reference point here, too, is the ASIS. Here it moves *up* and *backward,* while at the same time the ischium moves *forward.*

These movements are often proposed as preparations for delivery. However, anteversion **(1)** and retroversion **(2)** are movements at the coxofemoral (hip) level and not between the bones of the pelvis. *Performed in a moderate range of motion, they do not have any direct effect on the interior shape of the pelvis.* Rather, they can be used to guide the pelvis.

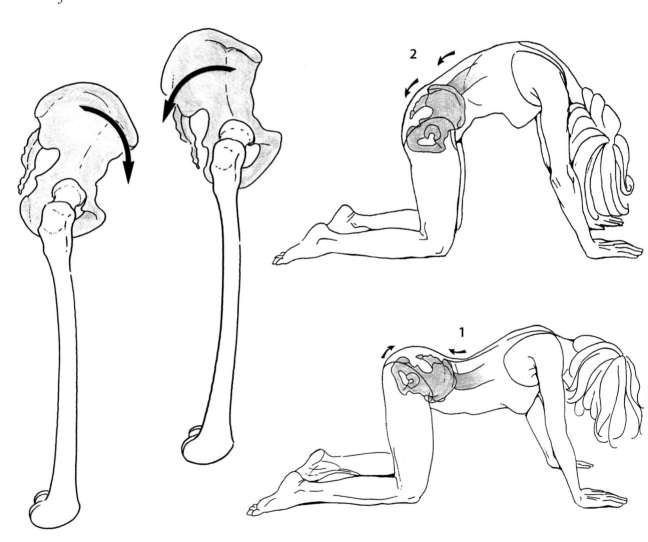

Movement of the Femur to the Front or Back
(Flexion and Extension)

On the inside of the cotyles, the femoral head can pivot from front to back, which permits movement of the femur into

- **Flexion** (to the front)
- **Extension** (to the back)

At the time of delivery, flexion is almost always in play, much more so than extension.

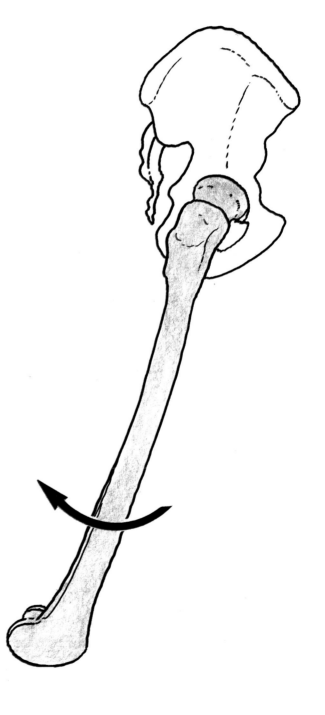

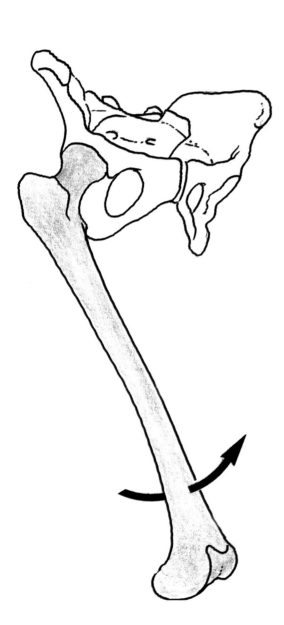

Frontal Movements of the Pelvis at the Hips:
Internal (Medial) and External (Lateral) Inclination

We look at only one hip when observing these movements.

Medial inclination of the pelvis is a movement that rocks the pelvis (as a whole) laterally at the level of the hips. The reference point is the ASIS, which moves *toward the midline* of the body, while at the same time the ischium moves *toward the outside.*

Lateral inclination of the pelvis is also a lateral movement of the entire pelvis at the level of the hips. The reference point here, too, is the ASIS. It moves *toward the outside* of the body, while, at the same time, the ischium moves *toward the midline* of the body.

Here, too, these are movements that happen at the coxofemoral (hip) level and not between the bones of the pelvis. *Performed in a moderate range of motion, they do not have any direct effect on the interior shape of the pelvis.* Rather, they can be used to guide the pelvis (see "The Pelvis Tilts," p. 146).

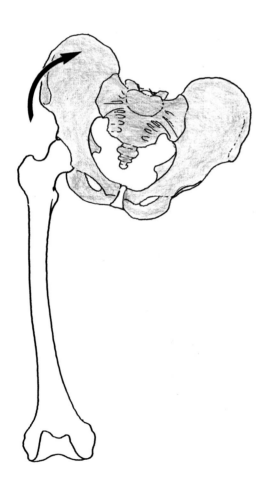

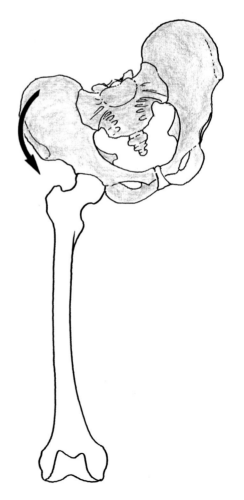

Frontal Movement of the Femur
(Abduction and Adduction)

On the inside of the cotyles, the femoral head can pivot sideways, which allows for lateral movement of the femur in

- **Abduction** (toward the outside)
- **Adduction** (toward the midline)

On Delivery Day

At the time of engagement, it is possible that both abduction and adduction can be seen (see chapters 7 and 8). At the time of disengagement, *abduction is almost always seen,* combined with more or less flexion (see p. 86).

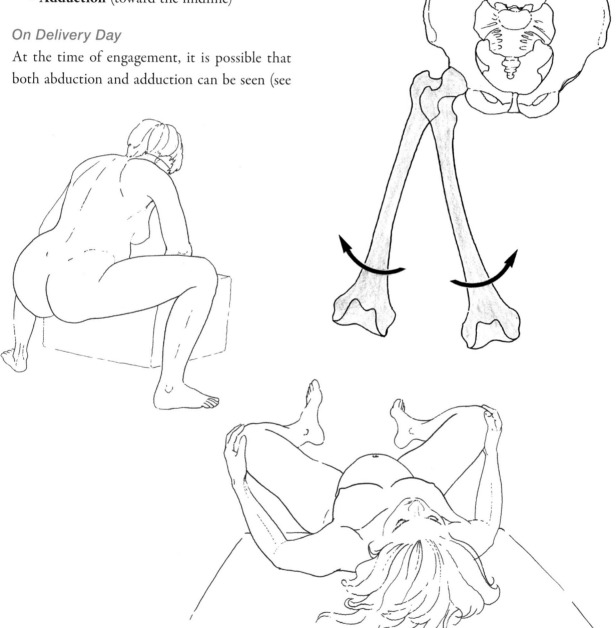

Transverse Movements of the Pelvis at the Hips
(Internal and External Rotation)

Internal Rotation

Internal rotation of the pelvis is a movement of the entire pelvis in horizontal torsion at the hips. The reference point is the ASIS, which moves horizontally *toward the midline* of the trunk.

External Rotation

External rotation of the pelvis is, likewise, a movement of the entire pelvis in horizontal torsion at the hips. The reference point here, too, is the ASIS, which turns *outward*.

Internal and external rotation of the pelvis happen at the coxofemoral (hip) level and not between the bones of the pelvis. *Performed in a moderate range of motion, they do not have any direct effect on the interior shape of the pelvis.* Rather, they can be used to guide the pelvis.

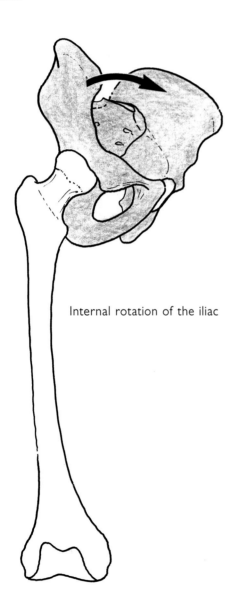

Internal rotation of the iliac

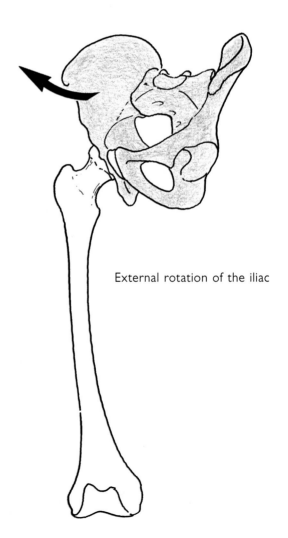

External rotation of the iliac

Rotation of the Femur

The femoral head can pivot on the inside of the cotyles, which permits movement of the femur (or femoral movements of the hip) in

- **External rotation,** which turns the thigh outward

- **Internal rotation,** which turns the thigh inward

At the time of delivery, rotation of the femur is often combined with flexion. At a certain amplitude, rotation of the femurs has an important influence on the form of the pelvic cavity (see pp. 90–93).

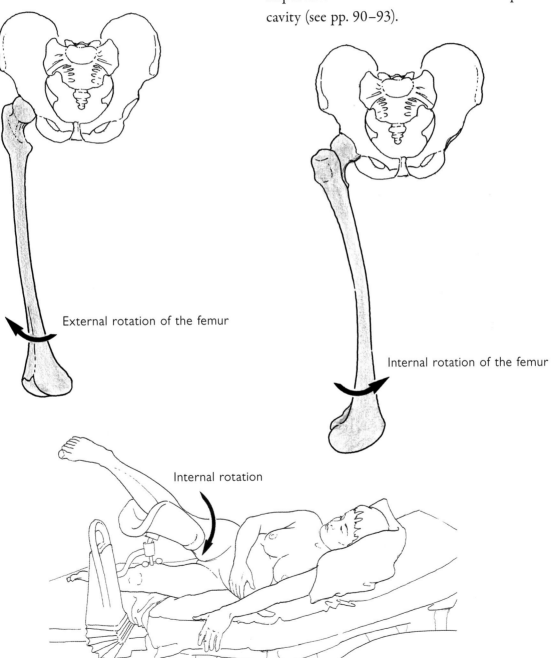

External rotation of the femur

Internal rotation of the femur

Internal rotation

Flexion of the Hip—
Method of Observation and Calculation

At the time of delivery, the woman's thighs are bent to a greater or lesser degree. We need to learn to evaluate this flexion visually, and rapidly, at the time of delivery and also during preparatory sessions. Why? Because depending on the position of the legs, the iliac bones are *freed up* (see "Unrestricted pelvis," p. 41) or *pulled into retroversion*.

If only the iliac bone (and not the whole pelvis) is involved, this is **iliac nutation** (see p. 46).

We observe the angle formed between the plane extending from the trunk and that extending from the femurs.

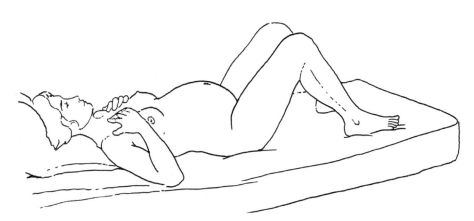

Here, with the legs slightly bent, the angle is 45°.

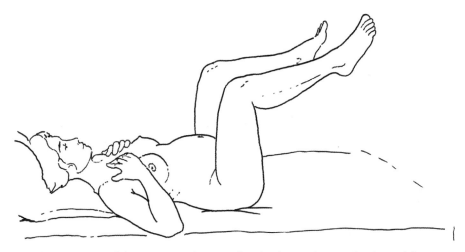

If the legs are bent close to vertical for a woman lying on her back, or close to horizontal for a woman who is seated, the angle is 90°. Until we reach 90°, the pelvis is "free" to bring itself into anteversion or retroversion.

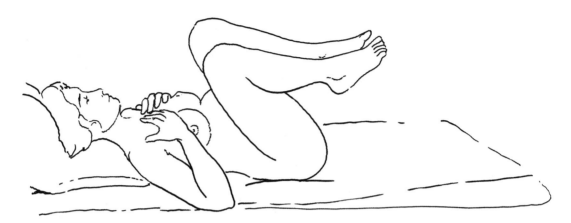

When the angle passes 90° (the thighs are greatly flexed), the pelvis is pulled into retroversion and the iliac bones into iliac nutation.

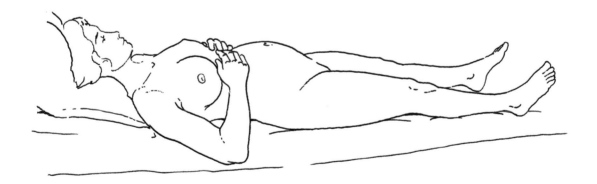

Here, with the woman standing, or lying on her back, with her legs extended, the angle is roughly zero (about 0°).

The "Traps" when Measuring Rotation
of the Hip in Flexion

Many situations can be misleading when we look at the direction of rotation of the femur.

When there is flexion at the knee, look at the foot.

- When it falls to the outside, the femur is in *internal* rotation.
- When it falls to the inside, the femur is in *external* rotation.

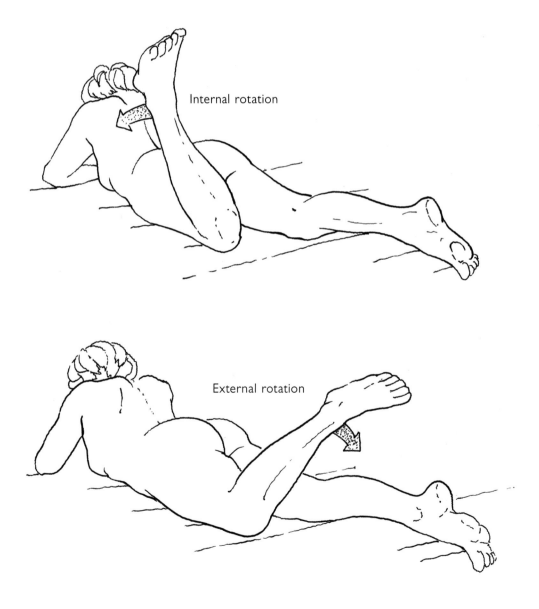

Internal rotation

External rotation

If the hip moves into flexion, look at the foot.

- If it moves to the outside, the femur goes into *internal* rotation.
- If it moves to the inside, the femur goes into *external* rotation.

Very important: when we flex or abduct the hip, we tend to automatically externally rotate it.

At the time of delivery, flexion is combined with abduction. Here, too, we need to look at where the foot is directed.

- When the foot moves outward, the femur goes into *internal* rotation.
- When the foot moves inward, the femur goes into *external* rotation.

See also the examples on pages 114, 116, 133, 137, 141, and 142.

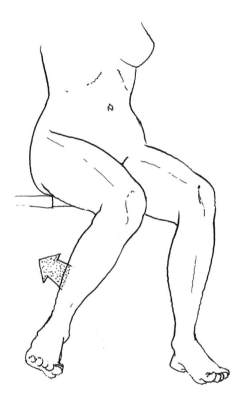

Internal rotation

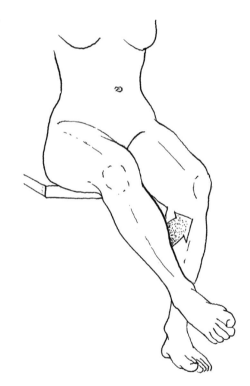

External rotation

5

THE PELVIS CHANGES SHAPE DURING CHILDBIRTH

How? Why?

Now that we have described the movements of the pelvis, we will explain what causes them. This is the most complex chapter of the book, and it is intended for those who want a deeper understanding of the movements. You can practice the exercises without having read this chapter.

THE PELVIS IS "LED" DURING CHILDBIRTH

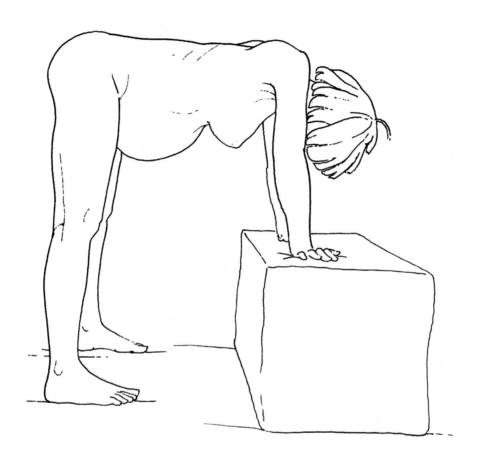

What Can Lead the Pelvis

What can lead the pelvis:

- The pull of ligaments
- The pull of muscles
- Muscular contraction

When in labor, the woman is asked to place her body in positions that are not normal for her, and in particular, positions that put tension on the "soft tissues": the ligaments and muscles.

When a ligament or muscle is **put under tension,** it pulls on the bones it is attached to. In this way tension from ligaments and muscles *pulls* on this or that part of the pelvis. This causes *intrinsic movements* in the pelvis and therefore changes its shape.

Traction on the bones of the pelvis can also come from *contraction* of the muscles that attach to the bones. This is infrequent in the context of childbirth.

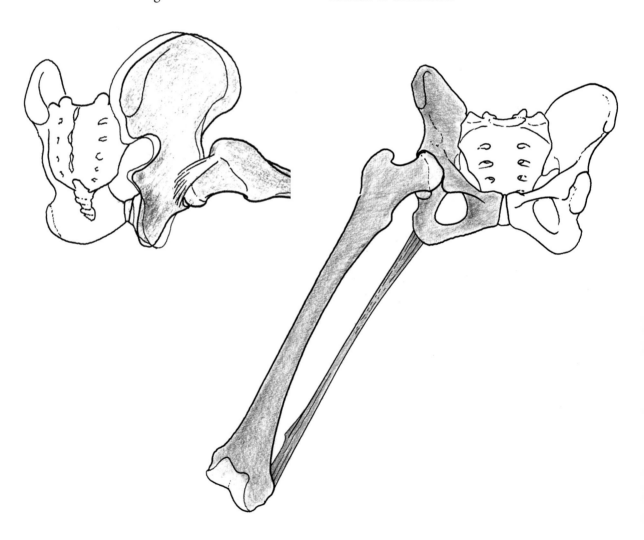

The Pelvis Pulled by the Spinal Column

Thanks to muscular traction, strong flexion of the lumbar spine pulls the sacrum into nutation.

When we take the spine into strong flexion, especially the lumbar spine, the **posterior muscles** of that area stretch, pulling on the back of the sacrum from top to bottom. They also pull the coccyx a little to the back and upward. This causes nutation of the sacrum.

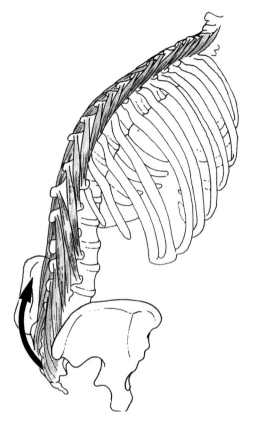

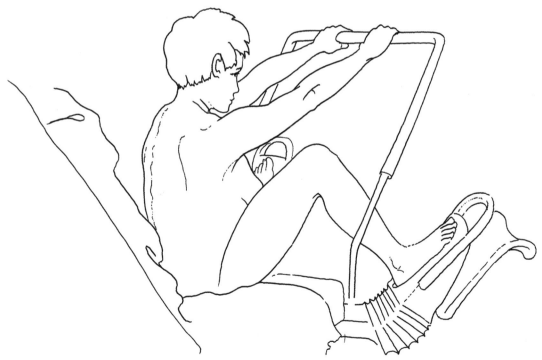

The spine can be brought into strong flexion specifically in three different positions.

- Lying on the side with the legs drawn up into fetal position
- Squatting, with the spine flexed forward
- Lying on the back with the hips flexed (if there is no pressure on the lower part of the sacrum); this is often the position a woman takes in childbirth: on her back, legs flexed in the stirrups, and the trunk in flexion

To summarize: Flexion of the spinal column contributes to sacral nutation from the outside. It is interesting to put this movement into play during the expulsion, for the final stage of disengagement, because it enlarges the inferior opening from back to front.

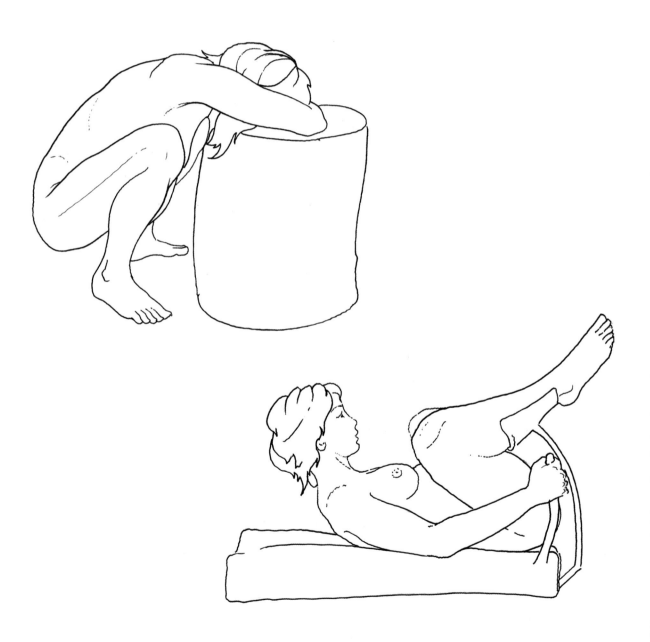

The Pelvis Pulled by
the Muscles of the Back

Contraction of the back muscles pulls the sacrum into nutation. The relaxation of the back muscles allows for contranutation.

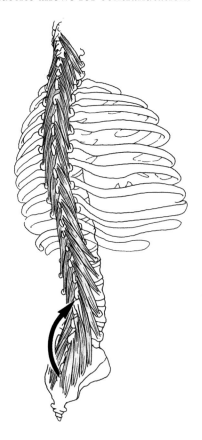

At the back of the sacrum and the spinal column we find deep muscles called the **transversospinalis group**. When contracted, these muscles arch the back and pull the sacrum into nutation. This contributes to enlarging the inferior opening and closing the superior opening.

Conversely, at the beginning of the delivery, during the engagement stage, the relaxation of these muscles allows the sacrum to move more easily into contranutation and permits the sacral plateau to move backward. This enlarges the sagittal diameter of the superior opening and facilitates the passage of the fetus.

See chapter 8 for positions that are specifically designed to relax the muscles at the back of the sacrum and allow the enlargement of the superior opening.

To summarize: Contraction of the muscles of the low back inhibits contranutation of the sacrum in the first stages of labor, in the engagement phase (passage through the first and second planes). Relaxation of these muscles is sometimes necessary to facilitate contranutation during the first stages in order to enlarge the superior opening sagittally.

The heat of a hand placed on this area can suffice to encourage relaxation of the transversospinalis muscles. This is simple and effective (see p. 156).

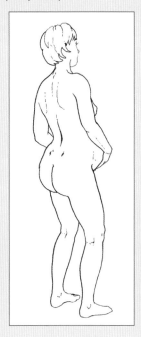

Abduction of the Hip = Adduction of the Iliac

Abduction of the hip initiates traction on the iliac, causing iliac adduction.

With a strong abduction of the hip, the inner thigh muscles tense and pull the ischio-pubic ramus.

- If the entire pelvis follows, we call this *lateral internal inclination of the pelvis.*

- If the movement leads only the iliac bone (and the sacrum does not follow), we call this **(1, 2)** *iliac adduction.*

The same effect is produced if abduction is combined with **(3)** a little flexion.

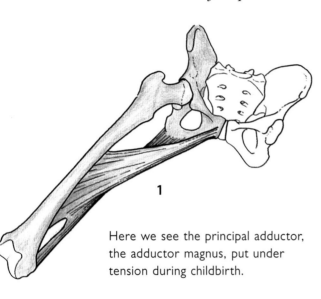

Here we see the principal adductor, the adductor magnus, put under tension during childbirth.

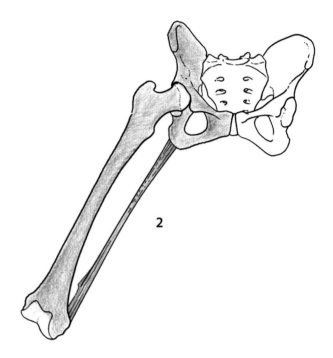

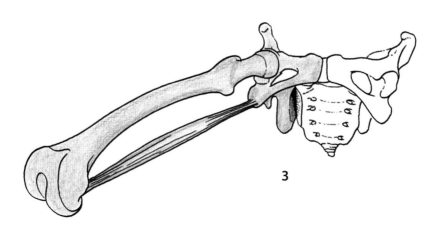

This movement, whether made on just one side or both, enlarges the inferior opening frontally (and reduces the size of the superior opening). Therefore, it is interesting during the disengagement phase. It is also vital during engagement, in alternation with the opposite movement, to help the fetus slip through (see p. 41).

(see p. 41)

We find the mechanisms described here at play in almost all of the final positions of labor. However, certain positions, such as lying on the side, will not accommodate opening the legs wide enough to pull on the pelvis.

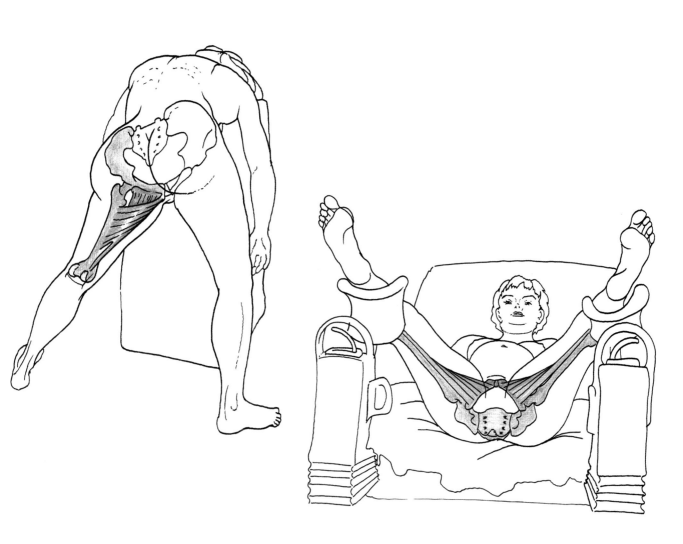

Adduction of the Hip = Abduction of the Iliac

Adduction of the hip initiates traction on the iliac, causing iliac abduction.

In adduction of the hip, its outer muscles—the **abductors (1)**—and the **iliotrochanteric ligament (2)** tense and pull the iliac bone.

- If the movement pulls the entire pelvis, we call this *lateral inclination of the pelvis.*
- If the movement pulls only the iliac bone (and the sacrum does not follow), we call this *iliac abduction.*

The same effect can be produced if we combine adduction with a little flexion.

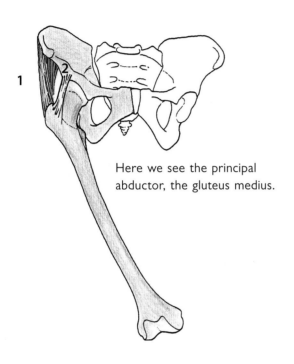

Here we see the principal abductor, the gluteus medius.

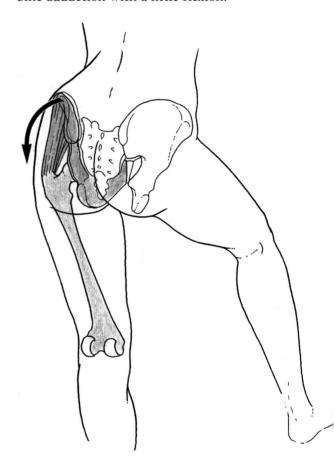

This movement enlarges the superior opening (and reduces the size of the inferior opening). This is interesting during the engagement phase.

During delivery we find this movement in the "star positions," in particular when there is transition of the pelvis. See chapters 7 and 8.

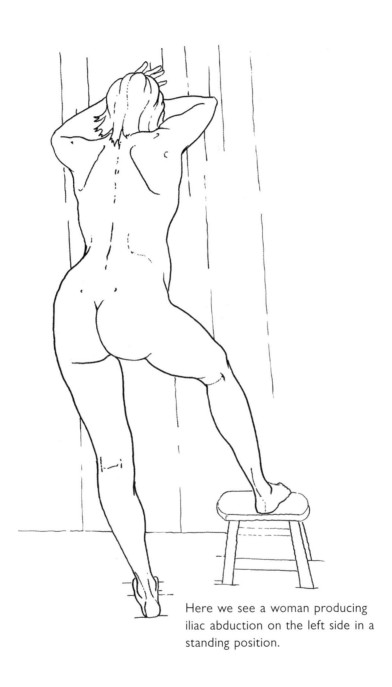

Here we see a woman producing iliac abduction on the left side in a standing position.

Internal Rotation of the Femurs and the Iliac

Internal rotation of the femurs causes internal rotation of the iliac bones and a separation of the ischial spines because of muscle and ligament tension.

When we rotate the thigh to the inside, the **posterior ligament of the hip** (not represented here) and the **external rotators (1)** tense and pull the iliac bones into internal rotation.

This movement opens the ischial spines. This is an interesting movement at the start of disengagement, during the passage through the third and fourth planes, even if it is done just on one side.

This internal rotation of the iliac bones has another consequence: the sacrum is less squeezed between the iliac bones and the upper part releases backward (sacral contra-nutation), which is interesting during passage through the first plane (the engagement).

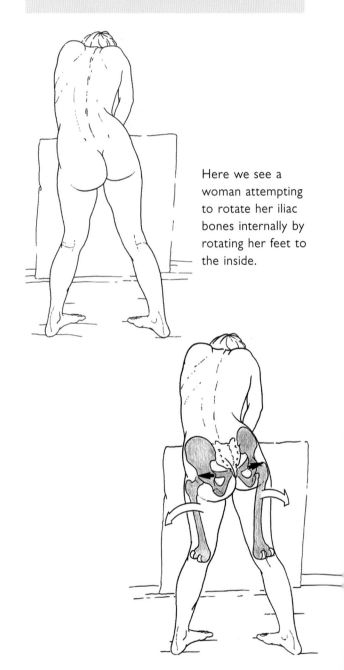

Here we see, among the external rotators of the hip, the posterior portion of the gluteus medius (at the top) and the quadratus femoris (at the bottom).

Here we see a woman attempting to rotate her iliac bones internally by rotating her feet to the inside.

At the time of delivery, we can create internal rotation of the femurs and iliac in a standing position.

90

External Rotation of the Femurs and the Iliac

External rotation of the femurs causes external rotation of the iliac bones and a drawing together of the ischial spines because of muscle and ligament tension.

When we rotate the femur externally, the **anterior ligaments of the hip (1)** and the internal rotators (not shown here) tense and pull the iliac bones into external rotation.

This movement draws the ischial spines toward each other. It is interesting to alternate this movement with internal rotation, to assist the fetus in slipping through the birth canal at the second and third planes.

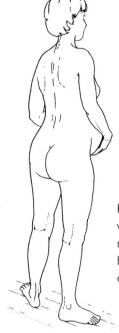

Here we see a woman attempting to mobilize her pelvis by turning her feet outward.

During labor we can rotate the femurs and the iliac bones externally in a standing position.

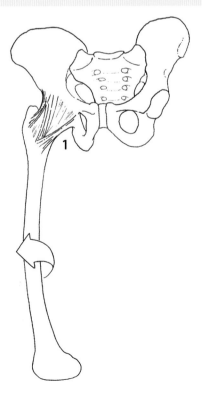

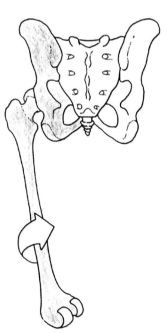

This external rotation of the iliac has another consequence: the sacrum is more squeezed between the iliac bones, which pushes the top part forward (sacral nutation).

Flexion and Internal Rotation of the Femur = Pronation of the Iliac

Flexion and internal rotation of the femur causes pronation of the iliac because of muscle and ligament tension.

When we flex the femur and rotate it internally, the **(1)** posterior ligament of the hip and one of the **anterior ligaments** (not represented here) tense and pull the iliac bone into pronation (see p. 62).

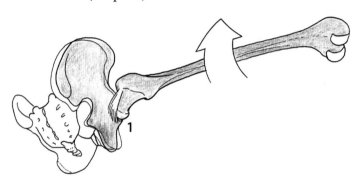

This movement separates the ischial spines. This is an interesting action at the beginning of the disengagement, at the level of the third plane, even when performed on just one side. We can find this movement in the "star positions" (see chapter 8). For example:

- Flexion and internal rotation while on all fours (see p. 133)
- Hips flexed in a standing position (see p. 137)
- Sitting on a ball (see p. 159)
- Squatting with the knees parallel and the feet separated (see p. 142)
- Lying on one side and internally rotating the upper leg (see p. 122)

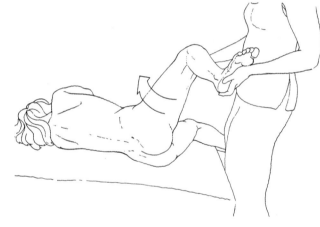

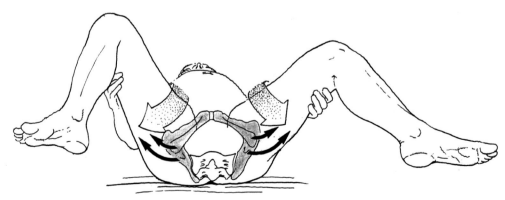

Flexion and External Rotation of the Femur = Supination of the Iliac

Flexion and external rotation of the femur causes supination of the iliac bone because of muscle and ligament tension.

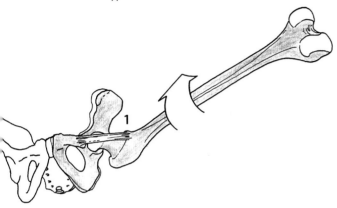

When we flex the femur and externally rotate it, the **(1)** pubofemoral ligament of the hip and the **internal rotators** (not represented here) tense and pull the iliac into supination (see p. 61).

This movement increases the span of the superior opening and, at the same time, brings the ischial spines closer together.

This movement is interesting during the engagement phase, even if it is done on only one side, especially when it is alternated with rotation in the opposite direction, going back and forth until you find the position that favors passage of the fetus.

At the time of delivery we find this movement in the "star positions" (see chapter 8). For example:

- Flexion and external rotation while on all fours (see p. 133)
- Standing with hips flexed (see p. 137)
- Sitting on a ball (see p. 159)
- Sitting cross-legged on a bed (see p. 113)
- Lying on one side and externally rotating the upper leg (see pp. 123–24)

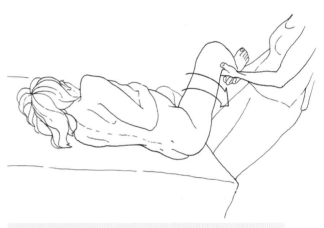

We often see women sitting Indian style, for example, in flexion and external rotation, when dilation begins (see p. 113).

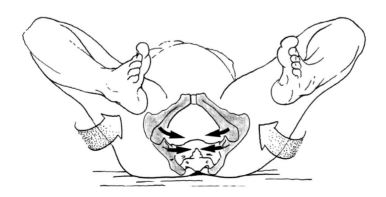

93

Hip Flexion and Iliac Nutation

Strong flexion of the hip causes iliac nutation of the joint capsule and the posterior ligaments of the hip and some of the posterior hip muscles, when put under tension, part of the gluteus maximus and gluteus medius (see p. 30), **(1)** the obturator internus, and **(2)** the quadratus femoris.

In flexion of the hip greater than 90°, the posterior ligaments tense and pull on the iliac bones, "ischia to the front."

- If the entire pelvis follows, we call this *pelvic retroversion*.
- If the movement pulls only the iliac bones (and the sacrum does not follow), we call this *iliac nutation* (see p. 46).

This movement enlarges the inferior opening sagittally (and reduces the size of the superior opening). This movement is interesting in the expulsion phase.

We can produce this movement in the following positions.

- Lying on the back, thighs in extreme flexion
- Lying on the side, hips in extreme flexion
- Sitting on a birthing chair with the feet raised high, causing strong flexion of the hips/knees
- Squatting

Note: in all of these positions, the knees are bent.

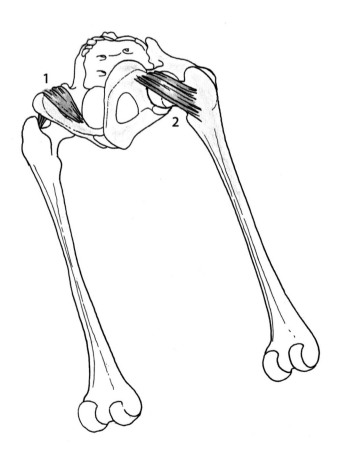

94

Hip flexion + knee extension causes iliac nutation. When we add extension of the knee (even incomplete) to flexion of the hip (even slight), we stretch the muscles at the back of the thigh: the hamstrings (see p. 30). These muscles pull the ischia forward, like the posterior ligaments (see top of pp. 120–21).

If you play with the amplitude of knee extension you may be able to reduce the amplitude of hip flexion.

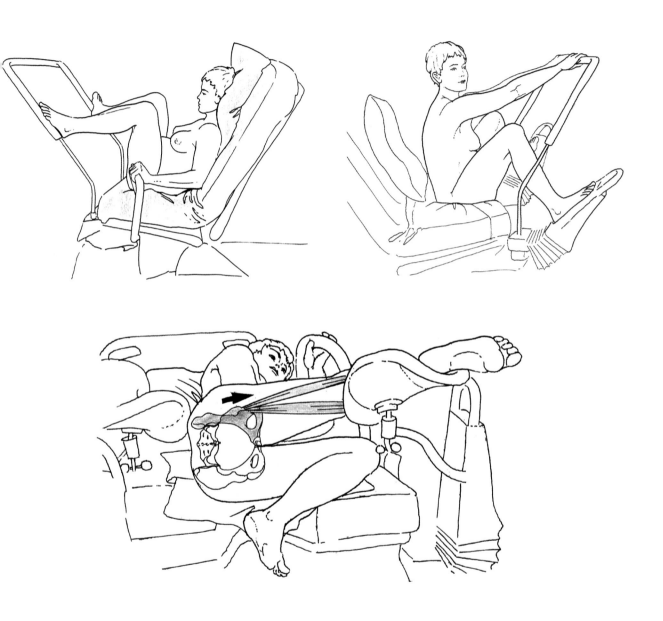

Hip Extension = Iliac Contranutation

Extension of the hip puts the anterior ligaments under tension, pulling the iliac bones, "sitz bones to the back."

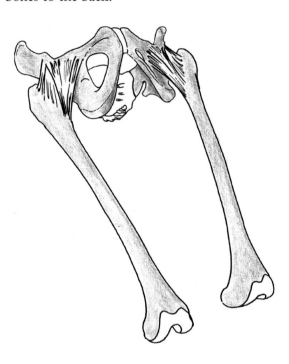

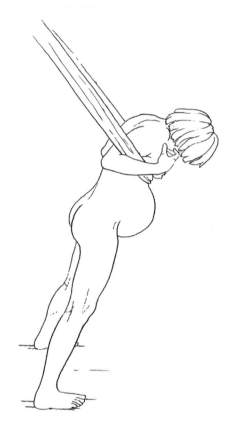

- If the entire pelvis follows the movement, we call this *pelvic anteversion*.
- If the movement pulls only the iliac bone (without moving the sacrum), we call this *iliac contranutation* (see p. 52).

This movement enlarges the superior opening sagittally (and reduces the size of the inferior opening). This is interesting for the engagement phase, or labor.

We can produce this movement in the following positions.

- Lying on the back with the legs stretched out on the same plane as the trunk
- Standing without the hips flexed
- Lying on one side, with the upper leg extended backward (see pp. 120–21)

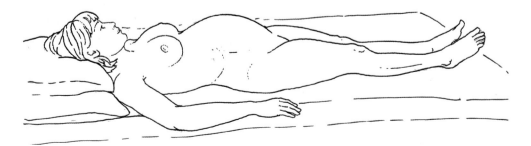

THE "RESTRICTED" PELVIS DURING CHILDBIRTH

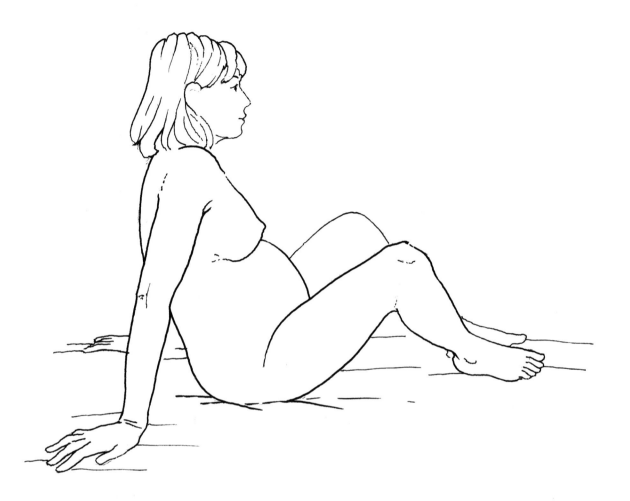

Pressure versus no pressure on the lower sacrum 98

External pressure on the ischium = abduction and supination of the iliac 100

Pressure on the trochanter allows for multidirectional movement of the pelvis 101

Support on a large ball changes pelvic mobility 102

Pressure can be applied to the pelvis through the femurs 103

Pressure versus No Pressure
on the Lower Sacrum

Pressure on the lower part of the sacrum produces contranutation. With no pressure on the sacrum, it is free to nutate.

If the lower part of the sacrum rests on a flat, hard surface (such as a hard mattress—see drawing at left—or the edge of the birthing table or birthing chair), it is pushed into contranutation, or, at a minimum, its ability to nutate is restricted.

Sacral contranutation (or impedance of sacral nutation) is interesting in the engagement phase, at the level of the first plane, because here the superior opening needs to enlarge from front to back. However, sacral contranutation is also involved during the disengagement phase. This is why it is important to ensure that, at these particular points in delivery, there is no pressure on the sacrum.

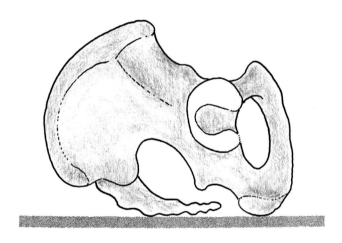

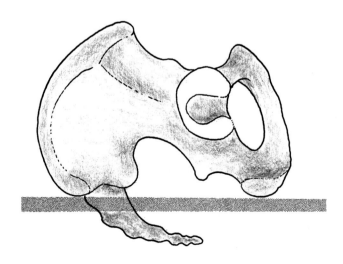

On a birthing table, we need to be able to get the part of the table that is putting pressure on the sacrum out of the way. If this is not possible, move the lower part of the sacrum off the surface that is restricting it, or place a malleable material (such as a gel- or water-filled cushion) under the sacrum.

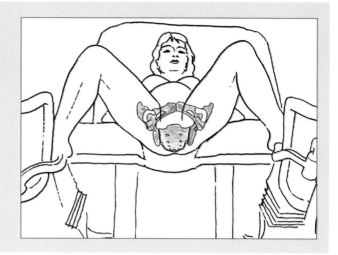

On a low birthing chair it is easy to become confused about sacral nutation, because the woman is sitting in retroversion. However, by positioning herself carefully, she can ensure that there is no pressure on the coccyx and the lower sacrum that would inhibit nutation. Any woman planning to use this kind of chair should practice on it before delivery.

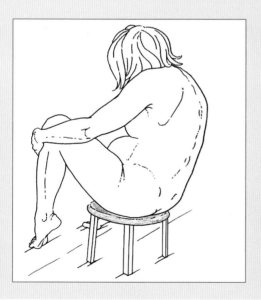

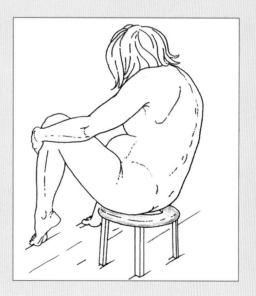

External Pressure on the Ischium =
Abduction and Supination of the Iliac

Pressure on the outside of the ischium causes abduction and supination of the iliac.

Sitting on a hard surface so that there is pressure on only one side of the pelvis pushes on the external part of the ischium.

As a result of this pressure, the iliac goes into abduction and supination (see pp. 56 and 61). This opens the superior opening transversely.

This movement is interesting in the engagement phase, when the fetus is passing through the first and second planes.

At the time of delivery there are a number of ways to create this situation of asymmetrical pressure.

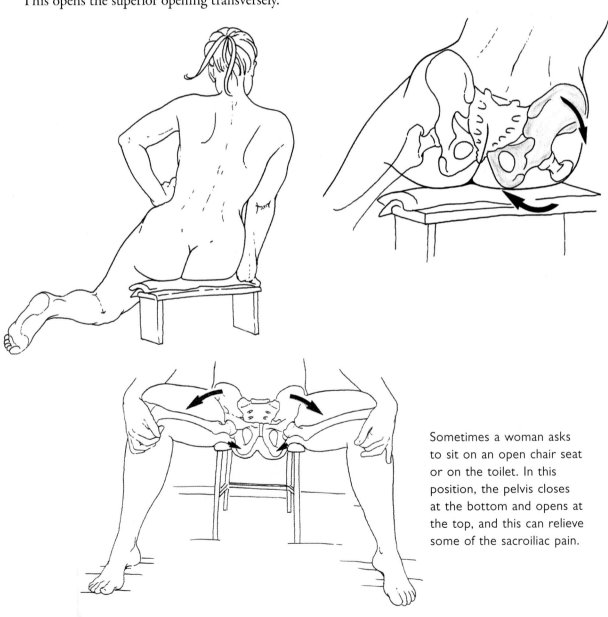

Sometimes a woman asks to sit on an open chair seat or on the toilet. In this position, the pelvis closes at the bottom and opens at the top, and this can relieve some of the sacroiliac pain.

Pressure on the Trochanter Allows for Multidirectional Movement of the Pelvis

When a woman lies on her side on a mattress that is relatively hard, she cannot put pressure directly on her pelvis. However, she is positioned on the upper prominence of the femur: the greater trochanter. This places pressure on the pelvis at hip level: the cotyle presses on the femoral head. Now this joint allows for movement of the pelvis in all directions.

This position is interesting when trying to mobilize the pelvis and orient it in all directions, including difficult moments when the fetus is passing from one plane to the next (for example, passage from the second to the third plane).

If the mattress is soft the iliac crest will also be in contact with it and have pressure on it. Pressure on the iliac crest will reduce the possibility of multidirectional movement for the pelvis, unless a malleable material (such as a gel- or water-filled cushion) is placed under the trochanter.

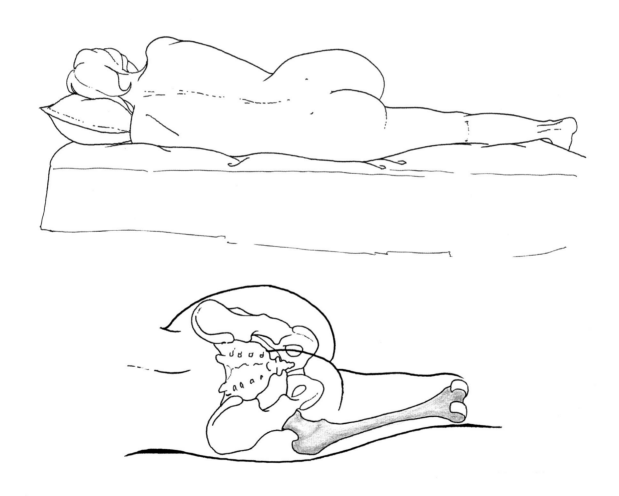

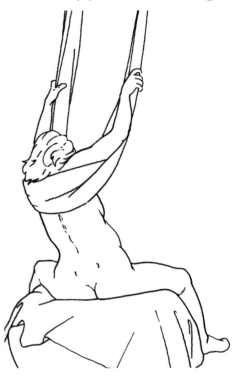

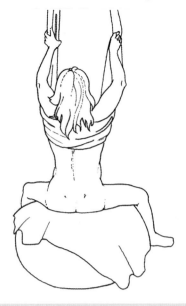

Today in delivery rooms we find large balls (60–80 cm in diameter) on which we have the woman sit.

A ball like this is not rigid and does not return the ground reaction force on the bones of the pelvis that a harder surface would, like in the situations described over the preceding pages. In addition, equilibrium changes from moment to moment, changing the way in which the pelvis is pushed.

This means that the pelvis is mobilized in random ways by the support. This change in orientation and mobilization causes, at the same time, the "sieve effect" and the "threading effect" (see p. 149).

We see such balls in use in delivery rooms as a means of facilitation, specifically for the engagement phase and the passage of the fetus through the first, second, and third planes.

> "I put into practice the advice given in the 'Pelvis and Childbirth' cycle with the women who come to our health center. They tell me after their delivery that one of the things that helped the most was moving on the large ball during contractions."
>
> TERESA MARTINEZ
> MIDWIFE, ALICANTE HEALTH
> CENTER, VALENCIA, SPAIN

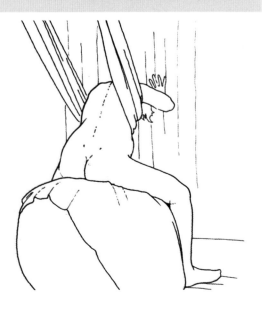

Pressure Can Be Applied
to the Pelvis through the Femurs

The femur, which supports the iliac bone at the cotyl, can also push back and change the orientation of the pelvis. We can compare this to the Chinese game of balancing spinning plates, where the juggler's stick pushes against and guides the plates. For example:

- Vertical pressure to the top of the cotyle orients the iliac in adduction (see p. 57).
- More oblique pressure toward the back of the cavity of the cotyle orients the iliac in abduction (see p. 56).

We can apply this pressure best while standing in a position with the knees bent or while on all fours. In these positions the pelvis is free to orient itself and be pushed on by the legs (with the knees straight, muscular tension does not permit this effect between the bones).

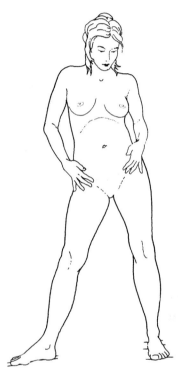

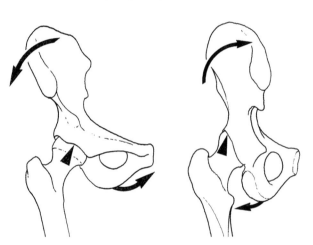

Here we can see that this standing woman is using her thigh to push her pelvis into inclination.

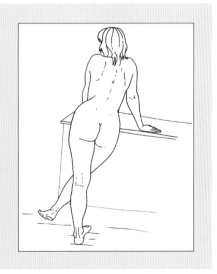

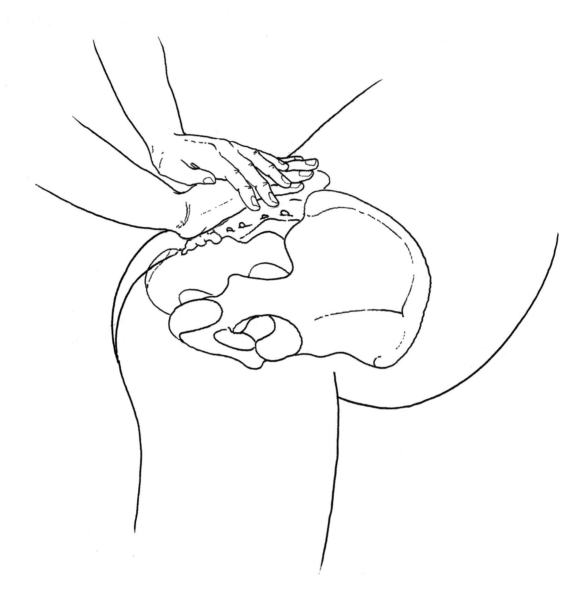

Manual Pressure on the Sacrum and Contranutation

Pushing manually on the sacrum can cause sacral contranutation. How can we do this without getting the opposite effect?

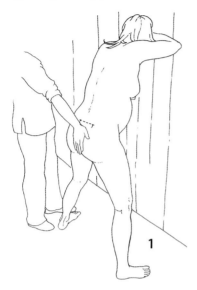

A manual push can tilt the sacrum. At the time of engagement we can do this and produce contranutation at the time when the fetal head is entering the birth canal.

> The point of pressure needs to be very precise: it has to be applied to the middle of the sacrum toward the sacrum-coccyx (**1, 2**), and not at the sacrolumbar level (**3**), which would produce the opposite effect.

The pressure needs to be directed downward and not toward the interior of the pelvis so that the sacrotuberous ligaments are not overstretched (see p. 20). The positions in which this is best performed are

- Supported standing (against a wall or some other structure)
- On all fours

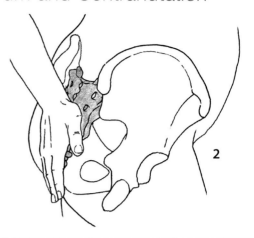

This manipulation was presented by Concha Cuenca and Pepa Santamaria, midwives at the Alcoy Hospital (Alacant, Spain) and analyzed in a workshop of "The Pelvis and Childbirth" series. They reported that they discovered this "push" just in time, when a woman was having persistent lumbosacral pain and the fetal head was stuck at the level of the promontory. They performed this action about three times during a contraction. The maneuver caused the descent to progress rapidly.

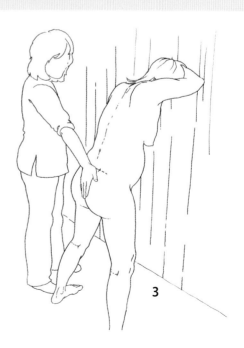

Manual Pressure on the Iliac Crest and Iliac Pronation

Manually pushing on the iliac crest can cause pronation of the iliac bone. How can we do this without getting the opposite effect?

By exerting pressure on the iliac crests we can mobilize the pelvis, pushing the crests closer to each other and opening the lower part of the pelvis.

Notice, however, that three versions are possible, with almost opposite effects!

1. If we push at the level of the tubercles of the iliac crests (see p. 6)

The movement creates *adduction* of the iliac bones. It separates the ischia, opening the pelvic outlet. This is involved at disengagement (third and fourth planes).

> The location of the hands is very important for this maneuver. It is preferable for people who will assist the woman at the time of delivery to practice this beforehand.

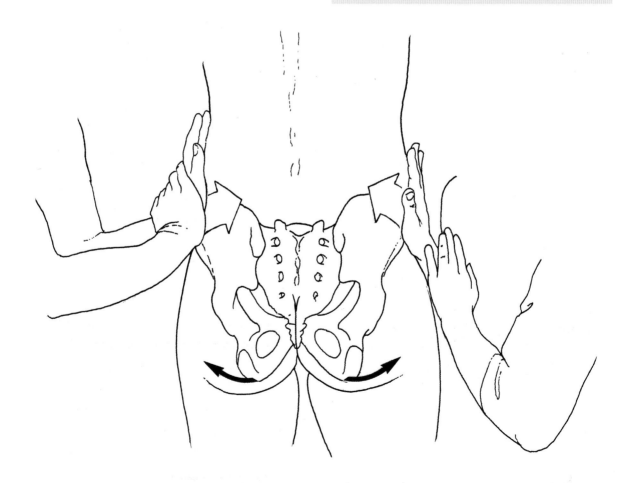

2. If we push in front of the tubercles of the iliac crests

Iliac adduction combines with a little *internal rotation:* we cause *pronation* of the iliac bones, which, in addition to opening the pelvic outlet, separates the ischial spines at the back. This movement is interesting at three stages.

- For the disengagement
- For passage of the fetus through the ischial spines
- For facilitating sacral contranutation, which enlarges the superior opening sagittally, which is interesting at the time of engagement (first plane)

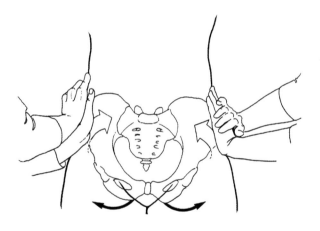

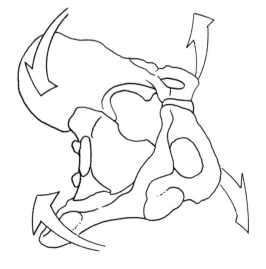

3. If we push on the iliac crests behind the tubercles

Iliac adduction combines with a bit of *external rotation:* we produce a sort of external rotation of the iliac bones. This does not open the pelvic outlet, nor does it widen the ischial spines. It is therefore effective neither for passage through the third planes nor for the disengagement.

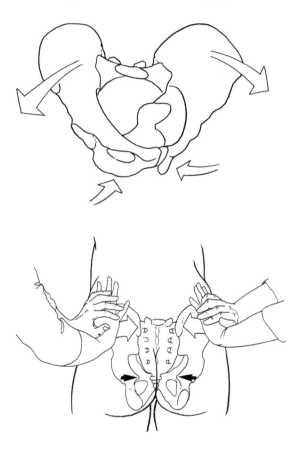

Manual pressure on the iliac crest to produce iliac pronation is a manipulation proposed by Ina May Gaskin, creator of the Gaskin maneuver, which is practiced in four-point position. For more information see the bibliography, particularly the article Gaskin coauthored, "All-Fours Maneuver for Reducing Shoulder Dystocia during Labor."

6

THE PRINCIPAL
POSITIONS
OF CHILDBIRTH

Introduction

In this chapter we take stock of the positions that are typically used today in childbirth. There are many other possible positions, and what we present here is just a small selection.

In the first positions presented, the pelvis is mobilized by the hips or the spine in a sagittal plane, that is to say, toward the front or back. These positions are shown in profile. They are simple enough to understand because everything happens on a single plane, and this helps in the first steps of comprehension.

The sagittal plane is the one in which the amplitude of movement is the greatest. Most of these positions are "classical": in a sagittal plane we can make great progress with these movements.

But, in fact, childbirth is an asymmetrical event when we are talking about the pelvis:

Positions are rarely organized in a *purely* sagittal plane. In practice they are most often combined, more or less, with other positions in other planes, thereby giving rise to many variations.

This chapter, therefore, proposes different positions in which we start with the sagittal and symmetric and then bring in the frontal and transverse planes, that is to say, hip rotation and the asymmetries of the legs.

This expands the possibilities and gives us the tools for analyzing what happens when a woman is in labor, when she is not limited in the way she can move and may, according to midwives, choose atypical or "bizarre" positions and movements.

These tools also offer the woman other possibilities for movement, helping her to understand why and how we use them.

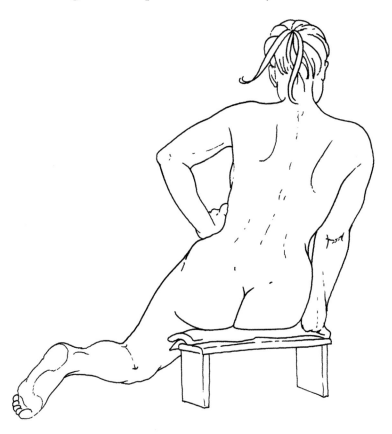

Parameters
of Observation of Positions

1. Description of the position

This is a global description pointing out characteristic components.

2. How are the hips?

Description of their position (see chapter 4).

3. How are the knees (and the feet)?

Description of their position.

4. Are the lower limbs symmetrical?

This is an important aspect to observe to see if the position corresponds to a possible asymmetry of the pelvis.

5. Is the pelvis under pressure?

This section describes which parts of the pelvis are under pressure and what exterior elements might be causing it.

6. Are the two iliac bones free?

Can they move, or are they in a fixed position or being pulled in a certain direction?

7. Is the sacrum free?

Can it move, or is it in a fixed position or being pulled in a certain direction?

8. Are the openings modified by the position?

Are they enlarged or reduced in size, sagitally and/or laterally?

9. Remarks

POSITIONS LYING ON THE BACK

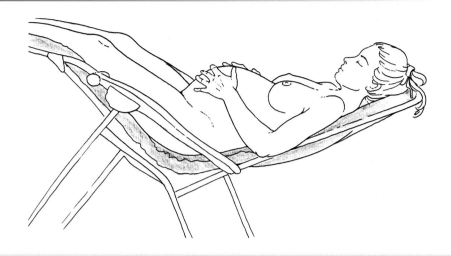

Presentation of the positions 111

Lying on the back with slight flexion of the femurs 112

Semi-reclining position 113

Lying on the back with extreme flexion and external rotation of the femurs 114

Lying on the back with extreme flexion and internal rotation of the femurs 116

Presentation of the Positions

We address the various positions of lying on the back first because they are the most common positions used in hospitals, particularly for monitoring, vaginal examinations, and epidurals. Numerous women also ask to lie down to rest when they arrive at the hospital.

If the fetus is already engaged (as is often

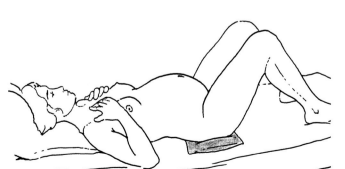

the case), gravity pulls it back toward the abdominal cavity rather than toward the pelvis.

When a woman lies on her back, then, uterine contractions must fight an uphill battle against two forces: gravitational pull that does not favor engagement and a lack of mobility of the sacrum.

In the event that this position has to be sustained during a gynecological exam, place a soft material—a packet of gel or water—under the sacrum so it is able to stay mobile.

In case the woman wants to stay in this position to rest, raise the bed so that the position of the uterus favors engagement.

Lying on the Back
with Slight Flexion of the Femurs

1. Description of the position
The trunk is flat, with the knees bent. The feet are flat on the bed or table, or in foot supports.

2. How are the hips?
The hips are in approximately 45° of flexion.

3. How are the knees (and the feet)?
The knees and feet are in about 90° of flexion.

4. Are the lower limbs symmetrical?
Yes.

5. Is the pelvis under pressure?
There is pressure on the entire posterior pelvis.

6. Are the two iliac bones free?
Yes, because hip flexion does not exceed 90°.

7. Is the sacrum free?
The sacrum is blocked by the bed or birthing table.

8. Are the openings modified by the position?
No.

9. Remarks
- Often women in this position complain of "kidney pain." The posterior sacroiliac ligaments are compressed. The fetus has to engage, but the position inhibits engagement, and this causes the pain.
- This position does not facilitate pelvic mobility. All of the posterior structures are restricted and compressed, and this can cause pain.
- This position is more practical for the obstetrics personnel than for the woman and is currently used during the engagement, especially in the case of epidurals and frequent monitoring.
- For the woman, this position does not require the work of any postural muscles, and it allows her to rest if she is tired. However, the contractions of the uterus fight against two forces: gravitational pull that does not favor engagement, and restriction of pelvic mobility.

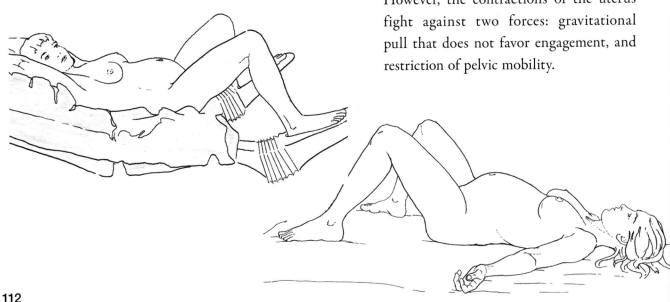

Semi-Reclining Position

1. Description of the position

The trunk is supported at an incline between 20° and 45° (either by a bed that raises or by large, firm cushions). The legs are stretched out, crossed Indian-style, or moderately bent at the hips and knees.

2. How are the hips?

The hips are positioned between 45° and 90°.

3. How are the knees (and the feet)?

The knees and feet are flexed to varying degrees.

4. Are the lower limbs symmetrical?

The legs can be symmetrical or not.

5. Is the pelvis under pressure?

There is pressure on the back of the ischia and on the sacrum, fixing the pelvis in retroversion.

6. Are the two iliac bones free?

The iliac bones can move at hip level.

7. Is the sacrum free?

It retains a bit of mobility. The pressure on the coccyx pushes it into contranutation.

8. Are the openings modified by the position?

No.

9. Remarks

- The extrinsic muscles of the hip are relaxed. Therefore the hip muscles do not restrict the movement of the pelvis.
- In terms of the muscles and joints, the pelvis has a lot of freedom.
- Although the pelvis is restricted by the pressure and supported from behind, it is pulled most often into retroversion, especially as the pregnant abdomen gravitates in the same direction.

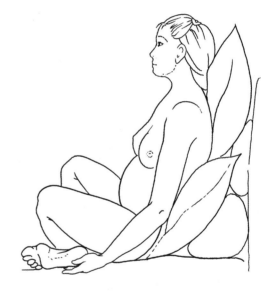

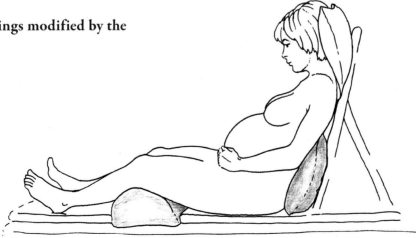

Lying on the Back with Extreme Flexion and External Rotation of the Femurs

1. Description of the position

The trunk is reclining, more or less supported. The legs are placed in supports in strong flexion, with the thighs in external rotation.

2. How are the hips?

The hips are in more than 90° of flexion, abduction, and external rotation all at the same time.

3. How are the knees (and the feet)?

The knees are bent and the feet are without pressure.

4. Are the lower limbs symmetrical?

Yes.

5. Is the pelvis under pressure?

The posterior side of the pelvis is under pressure.

6. Are the two iliac bones free?

They are pulled into nutation by the hip flexion and into supination by the external rotation.

7. Is the sacrum free?

It is restricted by the pressure of the table, unless that part of the table is removed.

8. Are the openings modified by the position?

The inferior opening enlarges from front to back and narrows laterally.

9. Remarks

- For many years this was the only position used during the final stages of labor.
- It is suitable for the disengagement because of the strong nutation of the iliac bones. The sacrum can be mobilized into

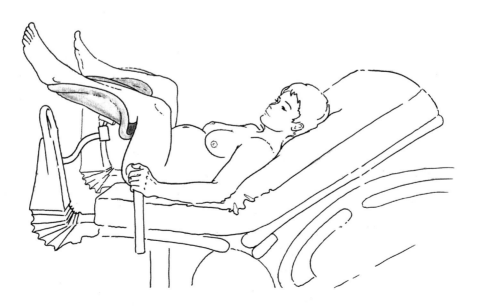

nutation by the fetal head on the condition that there is no pressure on it.

- In this position the force of gravity pulls the fetal head not toward the perineum but rather toward the back of the pelvis and therefore toward the back part of the perineum, which can become excessively distended (especially if the woman has had an epidural and is instructed to push with her diaphragm).

This position is less desirable in the transverse plane because the external rotation of the hips pulls the iliac bones into supination and narrows the space between the ischia.

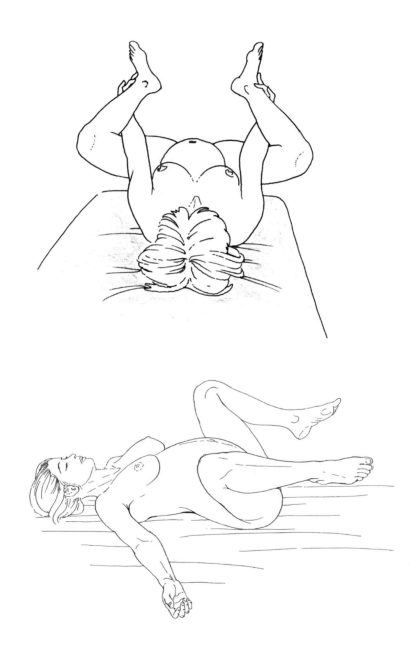

Lying on the Back with Extreme Flexion and Internal Rotation of the Femurs

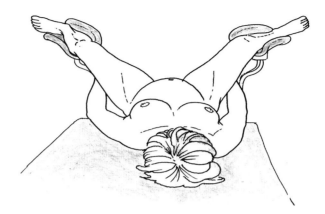

1. Description of the position
The trunk is reclining, and the legs are in the supports, with strong flexion of the thighs and internal rotation of the hips.

2. How are the hips?
The hips are bent more than 90°, with internal rotation and abduction.

3. How are the knees (and the feet)?
The knees are bent and the feet free.

4. Are the lower limbs symmetrical?
Yes.

5. Is the pelvis under pressure?
There is pressure on the posterior part at the upper end.

6. Are the two iliac bones free?
The iliac bones are pulled into nutation by the flexion of the hips and into pronation by the internal rotation.

7. Is the sacrum free?
It is restricted by the pressure of the table, unless that part of the table is removed.

8. Are the openings modified by the position?
The sagittal and transverse diameters of the inferior and middle openings enlarge. The anterior triangle of the perineum enlarges.

9. Remarks
- This is a position used in the disengagement phase.
- If the woman has had an epidural, the

This position is at once in the sagittal and the frontal-transverse planes, because the internal rotation of the hips pulls the iliac bones into pronation and enlarges the space between the ischial spines and between the ischia.

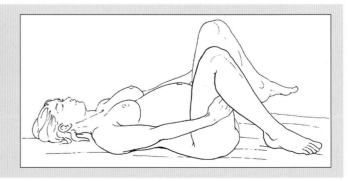

internal rotation of the femurs should be done very gently. If forced, it can damage the internal knee ligaments.

- If the woman feels like it, she can hold her thighs from the outside, which will bring the femurs into internal rotation.

Frog Maneuver

This maneuver was presented at a workshop by a midwife of the obstetrics team at the Maternité du Belvédère à Mont Saint Aignan (France). The team reported that this maneuver is effective in encouraging the descent of the fetus. The woman lies on the birthing table. Two people support her legs, one on either side of the table. Each mobilizes a leg at the hip, in opposite directions. Extreme flexion of the hip for one, and extreme extension for the other, external rotation for one, and internal rotation for the other, while moving in a circular motion in both directions at the same time. These movements pull the two iliac bones in all planes in an asymmetrical fashion. The pelvic cavity is transformed maximally. This maneuver can be done during the administration of an epidural and with the woman lying on her back.

POSITIONS LYING ON THE SIDE

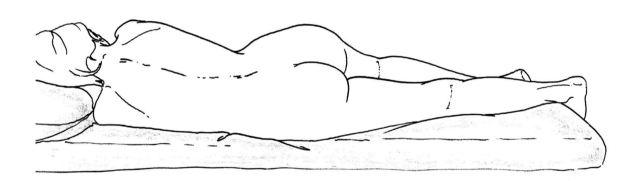

The positions on the side offer more advantages than those of lying on the back.

These positions are effective in all of the phases of the delivery. They can be held for a long time. The woman can rest and there is no contraction of postural muscles. The uterus is well oriented and often, supported by the bed, facilitates engagement in the superior opening, especially when an epidural is used. The contractions are effective, and the woman can relax while she is having them. Someone assisting the woman can massage, press on, or apply heat to the sacroiliac joint and the sacrum, which should provide some pain relief.

If the top leg is supported, the pelvis is free to move; it is not put under pressure because there is no weight on the top hip. This support allows the top leg to be aligned with the leg that is getting pressure from the table, inhibiting the adduction, which can sometimes hinder the sagittal movements of the pelvis.

This support also allows for many adaptations, which can facilitate engagement, especially in the case of an epidural: we can change sides and move the legs asymmetrically, creating numerous changes in the iliac.

The side positions are in the protocols of hospitals in the UK; in France, we often call them "English positions."

The variations in the upcoming pages should be used as alternatives and complements to the positions on the back during the disengagement phase.

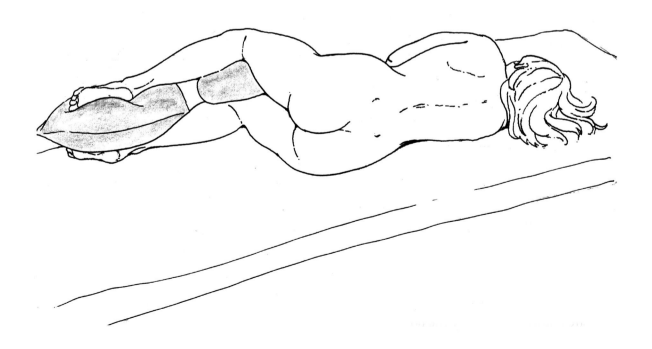

Lying on the Side
with Slight Flexion of the Femurs

*Also Called English Fashion
or Lateral Decubitus*

1. Description of the position

The trunk is positioned on one side, and the top leg placed parallel to the bottom leg, supported by a large pillow, leg supports, or a "hammock" system, or held by a third person.

2. How are the hips?

The hips are in flexion at about 45° to 70°, but not greater than 90°.

3. How are the knees (and the feet)?

The knees are positioned in about 45° to 90° of flexion.

4. Are the lower limbs symmetrical?

They are more or less symmetrical.

5. Is the pelvis under pressure?

The pelvis gets pressure at the cotyl, which is being pushed by the femoral head, which in turn is pushed by pressure on the greater trochanter.

6. Are the two iliac bones free?

The iliac on the bottom can be a bit blocked by the bed but still stay free. The top iliac can be moved in all directions. There is freedom of orientation.

7. Is the sacrum free?

The sacrum is free to go into either nutation or contranutation.

8. Are the openings modified by the position?

They are not transformed by the position. They are free to be modified by the fetus.

9. Remarks

- This is a position where the femoral head and the bones of the pelvis can adapt and work together optimally.
- This is a changeable position and can be held for a long time.
- This description is presented especially for the dilation period.
- This position can facilitate engagement at the superior opening, especially when the woman has had an epidural.

The upcoming variations are more suited to the disengagement phase. They can also be adopted intermittently to facilitate engagement.

Watch for tension in the lower back: the muscles have to stay relaxed so that the sacrum does not get fixed in nutation.

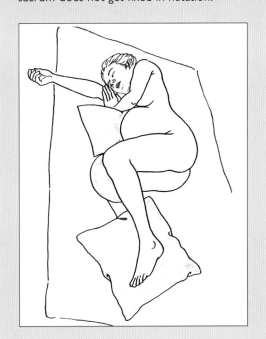

119

Lying on the Side with the Lower Limbs Asymmetrical

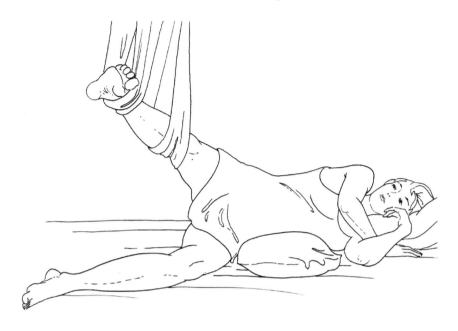

Variation 1: Upper Leg in Extension, Lower Leg in Flexion

1. Description of the position

The trunk is positioned on one side. The top leg is extended and held by a person or a support (fabric leg support). The lower leg is flexed.

2. How are the hips?

The hip of the top leg is in extension. The hip of the bottom leg is in 90° or more of flexion.

3. How are the knees (and the feet)?

The knee of the top leg is in extension. The knee of the bottom leg is in flexion.

4. Are the lower limbs symmetrical?

No.

5. Is the pelvis under pressure?

The pelvis gets pressure at the cotyl, which is being pushed by the femoral head, which in turn is pushed by pressure on the greater trochanter.

6. Are the two iliac bones free?

The top iliac is in contranutation. The bottom iliac is more or less free; it is a bit restricted by pressure from the bed up to 90° of flexion, and in nutation starting at 90°. The two iliac bones are asymmetrical.

7. Is the sacrum free?

The sacrum is a bit "scissored" by the position of the iliac bones, but all the same, the sacrum can be transformed from the inside.

8. Are the openings modified by the position?

The openings are made asymmetrical by the position.

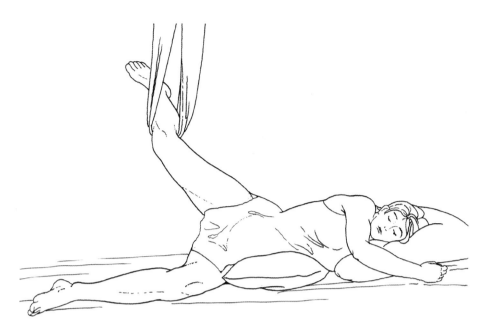

9. Remarks

- This position is useful when the fetal head starts to turn in the pelvic cavity, especially in the case of an epidural. For example, if the woman is totally dilated but the fetal head is still high, we will ask her to move the top leg—or the leg can be moved by another person—to mobilize the iliac and allow the fetus to slip through. At the same time the lower leg is free to move. In this case the pelvis can be transformed asymmetrically "in movement," as long as the woman alternates the position (variation 1 + variation 2) and changes sides.

- Testimonials of midwives say that here, the speed at which the head can turn and descend from the first to the third plane is spectacular, without the woman having to push too soon.

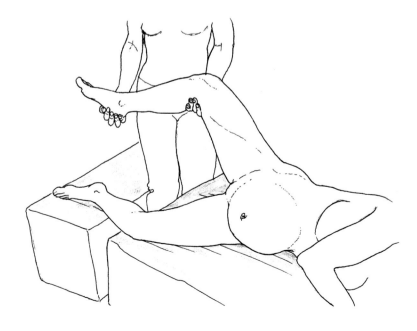

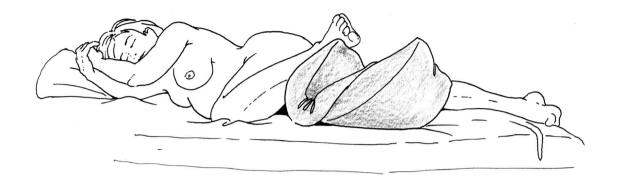

Variation 2: Upper Leg in Flexion and Internal Rotation, Lower Leg in Extension

1. Description of the position

The trunk is positioned on one side, tipped a bit forward toward the bed. The top leg is bent at the hip, with the knee bent and pushing into the bed. The top foot is raised and supported. The lower leg is extended.

2. How are the hips?

The top hip is in flexion greater than 90° and in internal rotation. The bottom hip is in extension.

3. How are the knees (and the feet)?

The knee of the top leg is in flexion. The knee of the bottom leg is in extension.

4. Are the lower limbs symmetrical?

No.

5. Is the pelvis under pressure?

It gets pressure at the cotyl, which is being pushed by the femoral head, which in turn is pushed by pressure on the greater trochanter.

6. Are the two iliac bones free?

The top iliac is pulled into strong nutation and pronation. The iliac on the bottom is pulled into contranutation.

7. Is the sacrum free?

It is twisted between the two asymmetrical iliac bones, which gives it less freedom of movement. Nevertheless, it is not restricted by external pressure and can nutate and contranutate.

8. Are the openings modified by the position?

They are made asymmetrical.

- **For the middle opening:** The top ischial spine is moved to the outside, up and forward. The bottom ischial spine is moved down and to the back.
- **For the superior opening:** The two ischio-pubic rami are asymmetrical. The one on top is moved forward by the nutation of the iliac and toward the outside because of the internal rotation. The one on the bottom is moved backward by the extension of the leg.

9. Remarks

See the remarks for variation 3 on the following page.

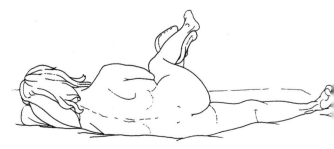

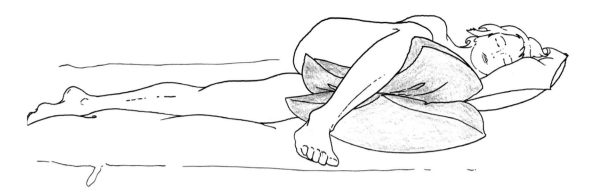

Variation 3: Upper Leg in Flexion and External Rotation, Lower Leg in Extension

1. Description of the position

This position is similar to that of variation 2, but here it is the knee that is supported and the foot that is on the bed.

2. How are the hips?

The top hip is in flexion greater than 90° and in external rotation. The bottom hip is in extension.

3. How are the knees (and the feet)?

The knee of the top leg is in flexion. The knee of the bottom leg is in extension.

4. Are the lower limbs symmetrical?

No.

5. Is the pelvis under pressure?

It gets pressure at the cotyl, which is being pushed by the femoral head, which in turn is pushed by pressure on the greater trochanter.

6. Are the two iliac bones free?

The top iliac is pulled into strong nutation and supination. The bottom iliac is pulled into contranutation.

7. Is the sacrum free?

It is twisted between the two asymmetrical iliac bones, which gives it less freedom of movement.

Nevertheless, it is not restricted by external pressure and can nutate and contranutate.

8. Are the openings modified by the position?

They are made asymmetrical.

- **For the middle opening:** The top ischial spine is moved to the inside, up and forward.
- **For the inferior opening:** The two ischia are asymmetrical. The top one moves forward (because of the nutation) and closer to the middle (because of the external rotation).

9. Remarks

- Variations 2 and 3 are very effective when the woman has had an epidural, and they are often recommended to women when the fetal head is still high in the pelvic cavity (first or second planes). We can ask them to alternate sides in this position.
- These positions are also used in all the phases of disengagement. There is maximal enlargement of the inferior opening, with several added advantages: on one hand, the asymmetry of the iliac bones, on the other hand, the sacrum being free. There are no restrictions in the back, and at the front the pregnant belly is pulled

toward the bed and away from the sacrum.

- These positions are comfortable for the obstetrics personnel, unless they're concerned about unusual orientations.

Midwives in Spain know this variation as the Sims position.

This third variation illustrates how just a small detail can change the internal form of the pelvis.

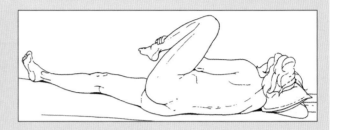

SEATED POSITIONS

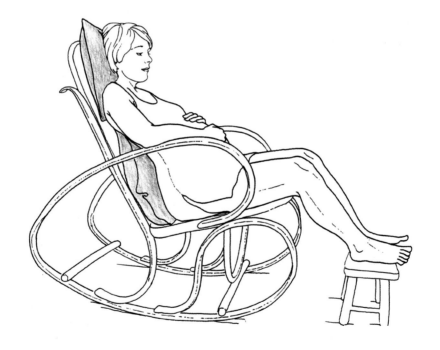

Seated Positions in Front of or Behind the Ischia (Sitz Bones)

1. Description of the position

The woman sits on a seat the size of a chair; it could be a couch, the edge of a bed, a rocking chair, stool, and so on.

2. How are the hips?

The hips are between 80° and 90° of flexion, depending on the height of the seat relative to the length of the woman's legs, and also abduction and often external rotation.

3. How are the knees (and the feet)?

The knees are bent. The feet are in contact with a support or the floor.

4. Are the lower limbs symmetrical?

In this position the hips are free, which allows for symmetry or asymmetry.

5. Is the pelvis under pressure?

The pelvis is under pressure at the ischia.

6. Are the two iliac bones free?

Yes, and even more so if the seat is soft and malleable.

7. Is the sacrum free?

The sacrum is free to move.

8. Are the openings modified by the position?

They are not transformed by the posture. It is the fetus that will modify them.

9. Remarks

Advantages

- In this position the pelvis can be "multi-positionable." We can constantly choose between anteversion or retroversion.
- From the point of view of pelvic mobility, this very free position should be used during all of the dilation phase.
- Gravity directs the mobile fetus toward the entrance of the pelvic cavity and works therefore in the direction of the uterine contractions. This favorable coordination of these two forces helps the labor progress.
- This is also a position where the femoral head and the bones of the pelvis can accommodate each other, enter into a

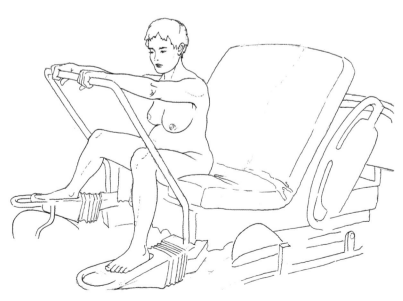

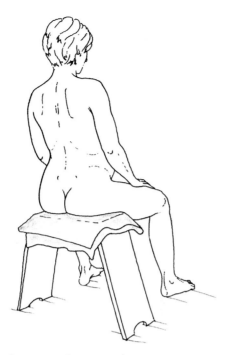

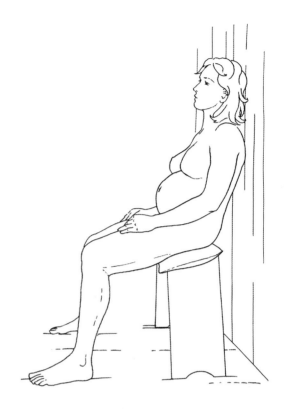

dialogue, adapt, and cooperate in an optimal way. The woman can also find a wide variety of leg positions, sometimes asymmetric.

Disadvantages

- This position demands that certain postural muscles work, which is difficult when the woman is tired.

- If the woman is seated behind the ischia, the sacrum is blocked. If she goes into anteversion by engaging the back muscles, this inhibits contranutation of the sacrum.

Seated Positions On a Low Seat

1. Description of the position

The woman sits on low seat, such as a stool or birthing chair.

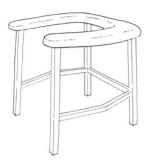

2. How are the hips?

The hips are in more than 90° of flexion, abduction, and usually external rotation.

3. How are the knees (and the feet)?

The knees are bent. The feet are on the floor.

4. Are the lower limbs symmetrical?

Yes.

5. Is the pelvis under pressure?

It is under pressure at the ischia.

6. Are the two iliac bones free?

They are affected by the pressure on the ischia. With pressure to the front, they are in anteversion, and with pressure behind, in retroversion. They are also affected by the hip flexion.

7. Is the sacrum free?

If the pressure comes from behind the ischia, the sacrum can be put under pressure and blocked in contranutation. If the pressure comes from in front, the sacrum is free.

8. Are the openings modified by the position?

This depends on the positions taken by the iliac bones and the sacrum (see points 6 and 7 above).

9. Remarks

If the woman is seated on a birthing stool, pressure on the sacrum from the posterior arc of the stool needs to be avoided so that sacral mobility is not inhibited (see p. 88).

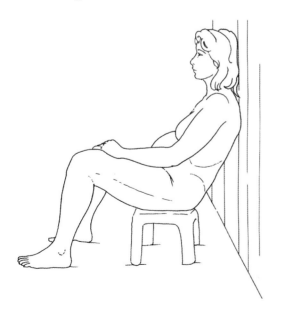

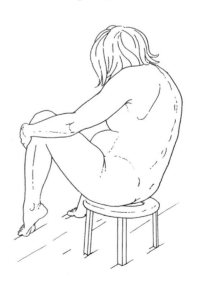

Seated Positions on a Large Ball

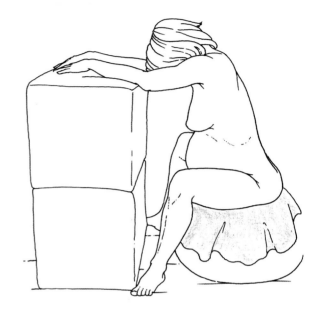

1. Description of the position

The woman sits on a large ball. Her trunk and arms can be placed on a fixed support (bed rails, the back of a chair, a third person supports the woman, et cetera). The legs can adopt many positions.

2. How are the hips?

The hips are in flexion between 80° and 90°, with a little abduction. Ideally, the woman chooses the size of the ball.

3. How are the knees (and the feet)?

The knees are bent. The feet are on the floor.

4. Are the lower limbs symmetrical?

The legs are symmetrical to start with. The more comfortable the woman gets on the ball, the more she can find asymmetrical positions for the legs.

Very important: if the pelvis stays fixed in anteversion or the back muscles contract (often these things happen at the same time), the sacrum stays fixed in nutation.

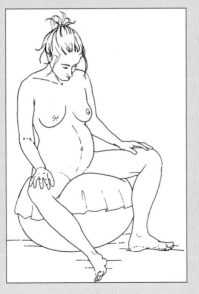

5. Is the pelvis under pressure?

There is hard pressure at the ischia as they sink into the soft ball, but the pelvis cannot be restricted because the support is very malleable.

6. Are the two iliac bones free?

The iliac bones are free to start with. The more asymmetrical the legs become, the more traction is put on the iliac bones.

7. Is the sacrum free?

Yes; this is a good position in which to let the sacrum nutate and contranutate.

8. Are the openings modified by the position?

The openings change shape with movements of greater amplitude (see chapter 7).

9. Remarks

- A mobile seat helps the pelvis orient itself in many directions.
- Making the legs asymmetrical, in internal rotation as well as in external, pulls on the iliac bones and renders the interior pelvis mobile from the outside.

- This position is recommended more and more at hospitals. It requires preparations to be made by the woman or midwife.

This position is thoroughly detailed in chapter 8.

KNEELING POSITIONS

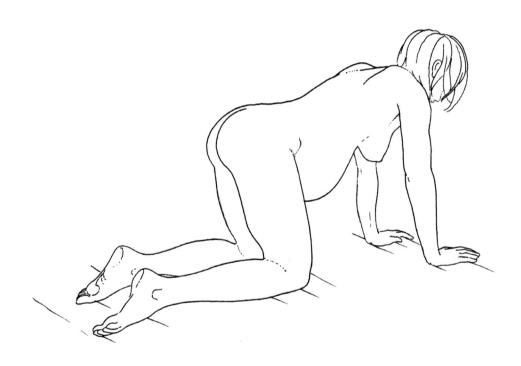

Kneeling Positions
with the Legs Parallel and Symmetrical

1. Description of the position

The woman has her weight on her bent knees and, more or less, on the upper part of her body (thorax, arms, hands).

2. How are the hips?

The hips are in about 90° of flexion (if the woman leans back, the flexion increases; if she rocks forward, the flexion decreases).

3. How are the knees?

The knees are in about 90° of flexion. As with the hips, the flexion increases or decreases depending on whether the woman moves her trunk to the front or back.

4. Are the lower limbs symmetrical?

Yes.

5. Is the pelvis under pressure?

It is under pressure at the femur heads. This is one of the positions where the pelvis is most free.

6. Are the two iliac bones free?

Yes; this is one of the positions where they have the greatest ability to adapt to the form of the fetus.

7. Is the sacrum free?

Yes, it can nutate or contranutate.

8. Are the openings modified by the position?

They are not changed by the position; they will be modified by the fetus.

9. Remarks

- Gravity pulls the fetus toward the pubis. This is not a position where the fetus engages a lot in the pelvis. If the woman has lumbosacral pain during labor, this position can help ease it, because the fetus is not putting pressure on her back.
- When the fetal head is already engaged, this position can facilitate progress of the fetus through the birth canal (as in the Gaskin maneuver; see the bibliography).
- This position is not used much by obstetrics personnel who are used to envisioning the fetus from a different vantage point, where the woman's pubis is facing up.
- At disengagement, this is a position where the pelvis can best adapt itself around the fetus.
- Starting in this position, a woman can easily find asymmetrical leg positions that suit her.

This position is thoroughly detailed in chapter 8.

> The pelvis is under pressure at the cotyls from the femur heads. No other part of the pelvis is under pressure. This allows the iliac bones to position themselves in all directions and the pelvis to orient itself in many planes. Here we can get the "sieve" effect (see p. 149). This position can be used in all stages of delivery.

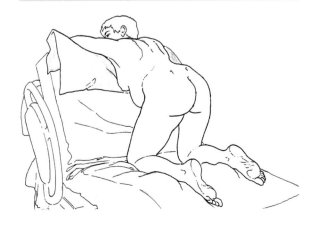

Kneeling Positions
with Internal/External Rotation of the Femurs

1. Description of the position

The woman has her weight on her bent knees and, more or less, on the upper part of her body (thorax, arms, hands). She adds internal and/or external rotation of the hips.

2. How are the hips?

The hips are in about 90° of flexion, increasing or decreasing depending on whether the woman leans forward or back. They are in internal or external rotation, or one in internal rotation and the other in external rotation.

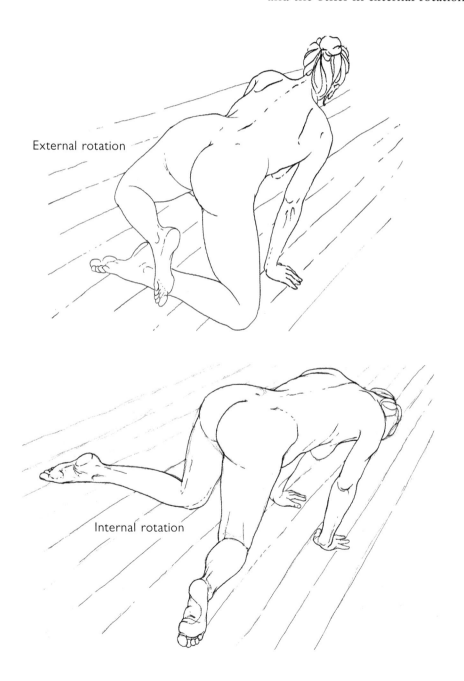

External rotation

Internal rotation

3. How are the knees?

The knees are in about 90° of flexion. As with the hips, the flexion increases or decreases depending on whether the woman moves her trunk to the front or back.

4. Are the lower limbs symmetrical?

The lower limbs are symmetrical or asymmetrical.

5. Is the pelvis under pressure?

The pelvis is under pressure at the femur heads.

6. Are the two iliac bones free?

In internal rotation the iliac is pulled into pronation. In external rotation it is pulled into supination.

7. Is the sacrum free?

The sacrum is twisted between the two iliac bones.

8. Are the openings modified by the position?

The middle opening and, even more so, the inferior opening are modified frontal-transversely: they enlarge with internal rotation and narrow with external rotation.

9. Remarks

When the woman understands the effects of hip rotation, she can use it to move the ischial spines and enlarge the lateral part of the middle opening.

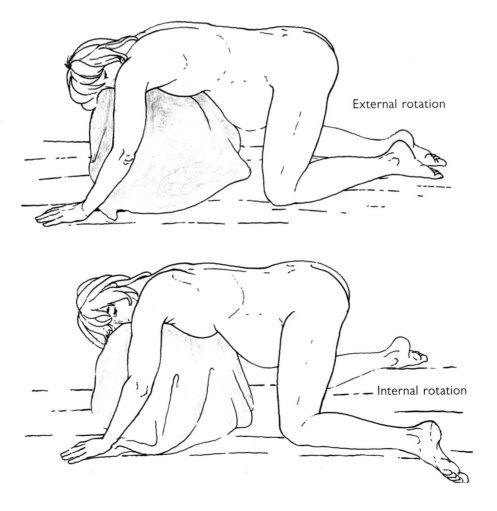

External rotation

Internal rotation

Kneeling Positions
with Asymmetry of the Femurs in Flexion/Extension

1. Description of the position

The woman kneels on her left leg, with her right leg extended forward and bent. She supports the weight of her trunk on her arms or a support. (This position can also be done oppositely, with the woman kneeling on her right leg and extending her left leg forward.)

2. How are the hips?

The hip of the right leg is in 90° to 120° of flexion, depending on the movement of the pelvis. The left hip is in extension.

3. How are the knees and the feet?

The knees are in flexion. The right foot is placed on the floor.

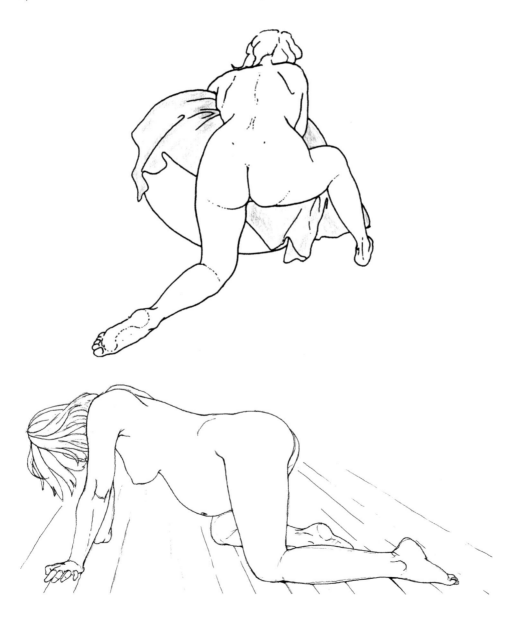

4. Are the lower limbs symmetrical?

The lower limbs are asymmetrical.

5. Is the pelvis under pressure?

The pelvis is under pressure at the hips.

6. Are the two iliac bones free?

The right iliac is pulled into nutation whenever flexion exceeds 90°. The left iliac is in contra-nutation because of hip extension.

7. Is the sacrum free?

The sacrum is twisted between the two iliac bones.

8. Are the openings modified by the position?

The three openings are modified asymmetrically. The right leg pulls forward the ischium, the ischio-pubic ramus, and the ischial spine on the right side. On the left side, they are pulled to the back.

9. Remarks

- The asymmetry of the pelvic cavity allows the fetus to slip through, especially if we alternate the position of the legs.
- Small movements (rocking, tilting, circumduction) encourages the "sieve" effect (see p. 149). Large movements encourage enlargement of the internal pelvis (see chapter 7).
- Many variations on this position are possible. If we alternate the rotations and the asymmetries, we discover how rich in possibilities this position is.

Everything that we describe here the woman can do spontaneously and intuitively, without instruction, if she is given the right conditions. It requires a calm and secure environment. Many midwives in our workshops tell stories of women adopting these "strange" positions on their own.

STANDING POSITIONS

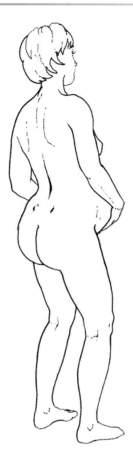

Standing Positions with the Hips Slightly Flexed

1. Description of the position

The woman stands, with her feet separated and her hips and knees slightly flexed. She pushes or leans her trunk and arms against a support (a wall, high bar, a suspended rope or piece of fabric, a third person, et cetera).

2. How are the hips?

The hips are in flexion from 20° to 90°.

3. How are the knees?

The knees are in about 20° of flexion, an important detail for maintaining a free pelvis.

4. Are the lower limbs symmetrical?

Yes.

5. Is the pelvis under pressure?

There is pressure from the femur heads.

6. Are the two iliac bones free?

The iliac bones are free to move; they can be mobilized from the inside.

7. Is the sacrum free?

The sacrum is free to nutate and contranutate.

8. Are the openings modified by the position?

They are not transformed by the position. They are free to be modified by the fetus.

9. Remarks

- The pelvis gets pressure at the cotyls from the femur heads. No other part of the pelvis is under pressure. This allows the iliac bones to position themselves in all directions and to have a lot of freedom regarding orientation. Specifically, in this position there is a lot of room for anteversion and retroversion.
- Gravity pulls the mobile fetus down the birth canal.
- From the point of view of pelvic mobility, this position lends itself well to all stages of birth, especially if the woman has learned how to move her pelvis.
- During labor this position can ease lumbosacral pain because it shifts the gravitational pull on the fetus away from the lower back (especially if the woman shifts her weight more forward on a support; see chapter 8).

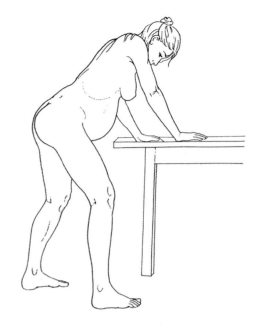

- At the disengagement phase this position allows the fetal head to slip through and the pelvis to adapt itself to the head, thanks to the freedom of the hips.
- This position is balanced on the back and legs, which helps prevent fatigue. The woman benefits from being supported/suspended.

This position is thoroughly detailed in chapter 8.

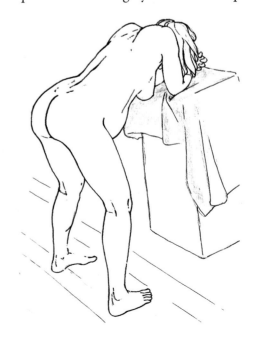

Standing Positions
with Internal/External Rotation of the Femurs

1. Description of the position

As in the preceding position (see p. 135), the woman stands with her feet separated and her hips and knees slightly flexed. We add internal or external rotation of the hips. She pushes or leans her trunk and arms against a support (a wall, high bar, a suspended rope or piece of fabric, a third person, et cetera).

2. How are the hips?

The hips are in a little flexion and in internal or external rotation, depending on what is comfortable for the woman.

3. How are the knees and the feet?

The knees are in a bit of flexion and/or rotation, matching the position of the hips. The feet turn inward or outward depending on the rotation.

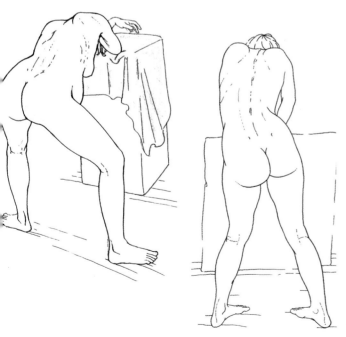

4. Are the lower limbs symmetrical?

The lower limbs are symmetrical or asymmetrical.

5. Is the pelvis under pressure?

There is pressure from the femur heads.

6. Are the two iliac bones free?

External rotation of the hips pulls the iliac bones into external rotation or supination, and internal rotation of the hips pulls them into internal rotation or pronation (see pp. 90–92).

7. Is the sacrum free?

The sacrum can go into nutation if the hips are in external rotation. Because of the opening of the back of the iliac bone, it is free to contranutate if the hips are in internal rotation (see pp. 58–59).

8. Are the openings modified by the position?

The superior opening is enlarged if the hips are in external rotation, and the middle and inferior openings are enlarged if the hips are in internal rotation.

9. Remarks

- When the woman is standing with her trunk vertical, hip rotation creates a "compression/decompression" by the iliac bones on the sacroiliac joint, which can relieve some of the ligament pain. This method of relief can be proposed to a woman, reminding her that it is she who needs to find the leg position that helps her most at each step of dilation.

Standing Positions
with Asymmetry of the Femurs in Flexion/Extension

1. Description of the position

The woman stands with her left foot positioned on a low support (such as a stool or footrest). She pushes or leans her trunk and arms against a support (a wall, high bar, a suspended rope or piece of fabric, a third person, et cetera). (This position can also be done oppositely, with the right foot on a low support.)

2. How are the hips?

The left hip is in a little flexion (about 45°, depending on the height of the stool). The right hip passes from extension to a bit of flexion. We could add internal or external rotation of the hips.

3. How are the knees?

The left knee is bent. The right knee passes from extension to a bit of flexion.

4. Are the lower limbs symmetrical?

No.

5. Is the pelvis under pressure?

There is pressure from the femur heads.

6. Are the two iliac bones free?

The left iliac bone is free as long as the angle of flexion does not surpass 90°. The right iliac bone is free if the knee and the hip stay bent, and it is pulled into contranutation if the hip is in extension.

7. Is the sacrum free?

Between the asymmetrical iliac bones, the sacrum takes a less frontal, more oblique position. It advances the side of the contranutated iliac bone, and it pulls back the side of the nutated iliac bone.

8. Are the openings modified by the position?

The openings are modified most when the right hip is in extension (see p. 153 and all of chapter 7).

9. Remarks

This position is interesting from many points of view.

- **Principal advantage:** The fetus can align itself and slip through the birth canal.
- Gravity helps with engagement.
- If we favor the right hip, the iliac bones are asymmetrical in the sagittal plane. It is interesting to experiment with amplitudes of circumduction of the pelvis (see chapters 7 and 8).

In this position some women ask for pressure to be put on the sacrum as the ligaments of the sacroiliac joint are put under tension.

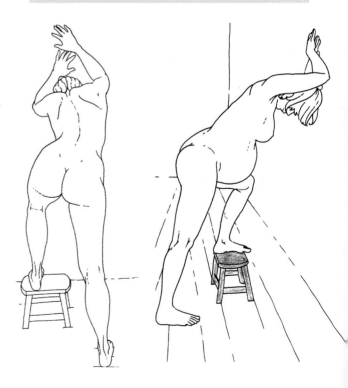

SQUATTING POSITIONS

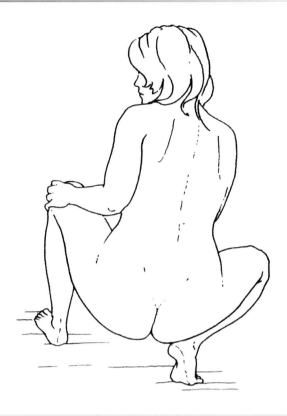

Basic Squat

1. Description of the position
The woman squats. Her trunk leans forward, and her hands can find an anchor (a bar, the end of the bed, a third person) if she likes. Her trunk can be supported or suspended with a sling.

2. How are the hips?
The hips are in maximal flexion.

3. How are the knees and the feet?

The knees and the ankles are in maximal flexion.

4. Are the lower limbs symmetrical?

Yes.

5. Is the pelvis under pressure?

No.

6. Are the two iliac bones free?

They are pulled into strong iliac nutation.

7. Is the sacrum free?

It is pulled by some of the spinal ligaments and certain back muscles into nutation (see p. 83).

8. Are the openings modified by the position?

Yes, especially the inferior opening, which enlarges sagittally in its anteroposterior diameter. The middle opening is also affected, but to a lesser degree.

9. Remarks

Many women who live in a culture where chairs are not used adopt this position spontaneously in the last phase of childbirth. Though it is not usual, this position could be adapted to the birthing table.

Advantages

This is a position in which the inferior opening is opened the most. There is a favorable coordination of forces: Gravity pulls the mobile fetus toward the inferior opening, moving the fetus in the same direction as the uterine contractions and orienting the fetal head toward the anterior triangle. The perineum opens dramatically; in fact, it can seem too progress too fast for some women.

Disadvantages

For a woman who does not normally sit in a squatted position, the position demands some work to stay balanced, which can be difficult if she is tired. Balancing can be made easier by a support placed under the woman's heels. She can also be suspended to lighten the weight on her pelvis and legs.

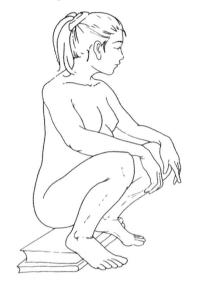

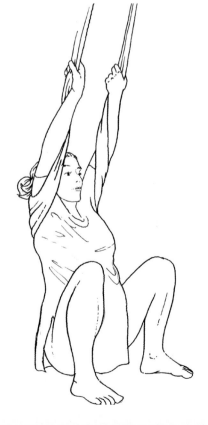

Squatting Positions
with External Rotation of the Femurs

1. Description of the position

The woman squats. Her trunk leans forward, and her hands can find an anchor (a bar, the end of the bed, a third person) if she likes. Her trunk can be supported or suspended with a sling. Her thighs are separated and externally rotated.

2. How are the hips?

The hips are in maximal flexion, abduction, and external rotation.

3. How are the knees and the feet?

The knees and the ankles are in maximal flexion.

4. Are the lower limbs symmetrical?

More or less.

5. Is the pelvis under pressure?

No.

6. Are the two iliac bones free?

They are pulled into strong iliac nutation with supination.

7. Is the sacrum free?

It is pulled by some of the spinal ligaments and certain back muscles into nutation (see p. 83).

8. Are the openings modified by the position?

Yes, especially the inferior opening, which enlarges sagittally in its anteroposterior diameter. The middle opening is also affected, but to a lesser degree. But external rotation encourages a lateral closing of the middle and inferior openings.

9. Remarks

In fact, squatting can never be assumed in the sagittal plane. Why? Because when the woman goes into strong hip flexion, her pregnant belly hits her thighs and she is forced to separate her legs. Thus, there is almost always an external rotation of the hips.

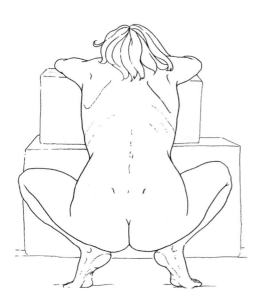

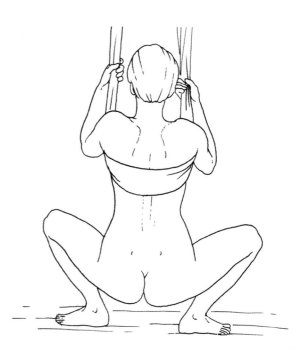

Squatting Positions
with Internal Rotation of the Femurs

1. Description of the position

The woman squats. Her trunk leans forward, and her hands can find an anchor (a bar, the end of the bed, a third person) if she likes. Her trunk can be supported or suspended with a sling. Her thighs are separated because of her pregnant belly, but her feet are spread farther apart than her knees.

2. How are the hips?

The hips are in maximal flexion, abduction, and internal rotation.

3. How are the knees and the feet?

The knees and the ankles are in maximal flexion.

4. Are the lower limbs symmetrical?

More or less.

5. Is the pelvis under pressure?

No.

6. Are the two iliac bones free?

They are pulled into strong iliac nutation with pronation.

7. Is the sacrum free?

It is pulled by some of the spinal ligaments and certain back muscles into nutation (see p. 83).

8. Are the openings modified by the position?

Yes, especially the inferior opening, which enlarges sagittally in its anteroposterior diameter. The middle opening is also affected, but to a lesser degree. But internal rotation encourages a lateral opening of the middle and inferior openings.

9. Remarks

Keep the knees aligned with the feet and the feet parallel to modify the orientation of the iliac bones, which are being pulled into pronation, laterally opening the space between the ischial spines and the ischia.

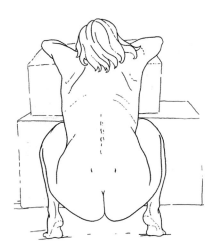

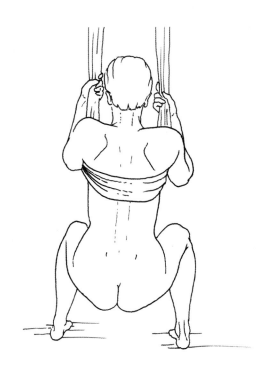

Kabyle Position

This position was transmitted to us by Dr. Nicole Ferry by way of an ethnographic document that she wrote on childbirth in Kabylie, Algeria.

Description

The woman and the midwife face each other. The woman squats on the floor, with her feet parallel (more or less, depending on what she can do). She places her arms around the midwife's neck or, better, grips the midwife's shoulders with her hands. The midwife places her hands on the woman's knees.

When the midwife leans back, she takes the woman's trunk into forward flexion. She can regulate the amount of flexion. When she pushes against the woman's knees, the midwife causes greater hip flexion, which encourages iliac nutation (from ligament tension, muscles at the back of the hips, and the gluteus maximus and gluteus medius; see p. 94). The midwife can, with her push, regulate the amplitude of iliac nutation, which opens the inferior opening. At disengagement, with no pressure on the sacrum, the mobile fetus will push the coccyx backward: nutation by pressure from the fetus.

This maneuver is particularly effective during the disengagement phase. In effect we see that the pelvis places itself in a "dropped jaw" position for three reasons: flexion of the trunk, flexion of the hips, and pressure of the mobile fetus. We can see here how these factors favor the birth of the child.

Variations on the Birthing Bed, with the Bar

The woman squats on the bed. She leans slightly forward to meet the bar, which she can lean on or pull on. The bar is pulled slightly to the front. The midwife is at the end of the bed. She places her hands on the woman's knees, as in the above description. The same regulation of the movement is possible.

Disadvantages

- The position crushes the leg muscles (bad in the case of varicose veins).
- Strong lumbopelvic kyphosis can cause or reawaken sciatica or lumbago. We prefer that the woman be more suspended to reduce trunk flexion.

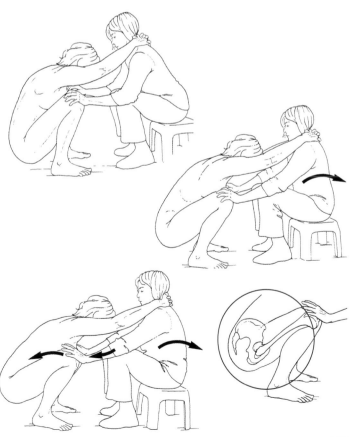

Marina Lembo's "Duck Walk" Maneuver

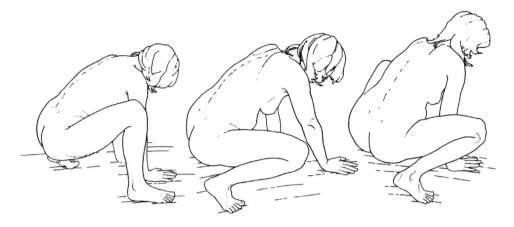

This position was given to us by a midwife in Argentina (Marina Lembo, who translated Ina May Gaskin's work into Spanish). It was analyzed by a group of midwives who were following our workshop series in Uruguay.

Description

The woman squats on the floor. Her hands are placed on the floor or on her knees, or they are held up by the midwife.

The woman starts to shift her body weight to the right, onto the right foot, then to the left, and onto that foot, as she "walks" forward in this squatting position.

Consequences

The weight of the trunk directing pressure toward the bottom of the pelvis and the asymmetrical movement of the legs imposing asymmetrical movement on the iliac bones at each

"step" move the pelvis intrinsically in such a way that it guides the fetus to the outlet.

If the woman has limited flexion in her hips, knees, or ankles, this maneuver can be uncomfortable or inappropriate.

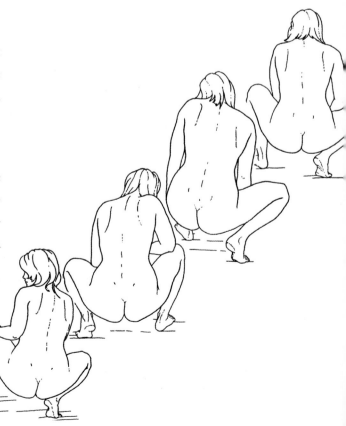

7

THE MOVEMENTS AND TRANSFORMATIONS OF THE PELVIS

This chapter looks at the most common pelvic movements a woman can make during childbirth and the consequences for the progression of the fetus. This subject is covered more extensively in professional texts (see pp. 167–69).

PELVIC MOVEMENTS
WITH A SMALL RANGE OF MOTION

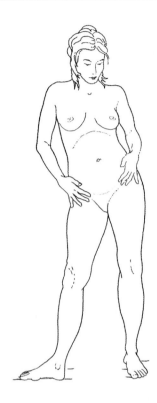

The Pelvis Tilts on the Femur Heads

We can make the pelvis tilt by maneuvering the hip joints and the lumbar spine, with the knees and the ankles adapting to the movement. The amplitude of this movement is very small, and consequently the pelvis is unrestricted (see the definition of an unrestricted pelvis on p. 41).

The pelvis can tilt into anteversion, retro-version, or lateral inclination (lateroversion) and into internal or external rotation (see pp. 58–59). All these movements are combined in **circum-duction:** circular displacement in all directions. We might call this swaying, swinging, or rock-ing the pelvis. We imagine drawing circles on the ground or behind us with the ASIS, the coccyx, or one of the ischia. Or we can draw a figure eight with one side of the pelvis or the other.

The desired effect of these movements is to change the orientation of the openings, specifically the superior opening, and to play with the relationship between the opening and gravity—which always directs the fetus downward toward the lesser pelvis.

In lateroversion the fetal head falls toward the innominate line of the side that is lower, which can help it turn and get better oriented before passage through the first plane.

In anteversion the fetus falls toward the front of the superior opening, which can be useful for freeing the promontory during passage through the first plane.

In retroversion the fetal head does the opposite: it falls toward the back of the superior opening, toward the concavity of the back surface of the sacrum, which can help confirm engagement, for passage from the first to second plane.

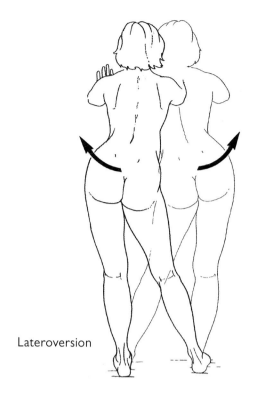

Lateroversion

In circumduction the fetal head does a combination of all of these movements. It "falls" successively to each of the bones of the pelvic cavity in a random fashion. This is adaptability in a broad sense.

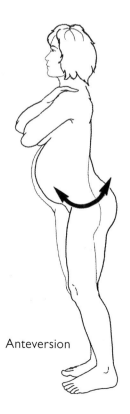

Anteversion

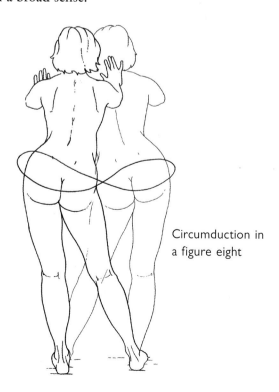

Circumduction in a figure eight

147

The Pelvis Transitions from Side to Side, to the Front, to the Back, and in Circles

We can move the pelvis while keeping it oriented in the same plane as the surface on which we put pressure (the floor, for example). These movements are called transitions, and they push the pelvis to the front, to the back, from side to side, or in circles. They do not change the orientation of the opening significantly.

Transitioning the pelvis creates a discrepancy between the alignment of the pelvis and abdomen, which are no longer superimposed. The part of the fetus that is still abdominal holds back slightly the part that is already in the pelvis.

If the pelvis transitions to the right, the fetal body stays in the left side of the abdomen, and the fetal head is a little less attached to the wall of the superior opening.

If the pelvis transitions to the front, the fetal body stays to the back and the head disengages a little from the sacrum.

These effects are minimal, but when the woman can connect transitions with the following movements, the pelvis is less static and the fetus can slip through more easily.

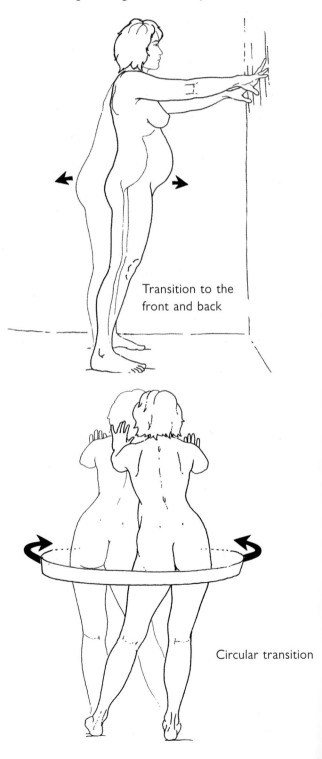

Transition to the front and back

Lateral transition

Circular transition

148

The Pelvis Tilts and Transitions at the Same Time

Often, in fact, we combine the movements of tilting and transitioning, which produces a double effect for the fetus: simultaneously, we direct fetal movement toward certain internal surfaces of the iliac bones and sacrum and away from others.

This is the "sieve effect" in its complete form (see below).

These movements, which are designed to aid the fetus, are also very effective for easing pain. Midwives report that when a woman practices pelvic tilting and transition, the dilation process progresses more positively, specifically in cases of asynclitism.

The "Slip" Effect

Movements among the three large bones of the pelvis bring changes to the dynamic form of the birth canal that allow the fetus to search for or find a way to pass through. This is what we call "slipping."

The "Sieve" Effect

The tilting and transition movements described at the beginning of this chapter both contribute to mobilizing and orienting the fetal head. We call this the "sieve" effect, because we have to think of moving the pelvis in the same way that we might maneuver a sieve to allow grains to pass through.

In doing so the woman allows her pelvis to adopt orientations that facilitate the movement of the fetus at each step of delivery. This "sieve" effect is used in passage through the first, second, and third planes.

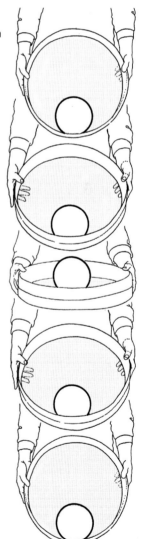

The pelvis tips in anteversion and retroversion.

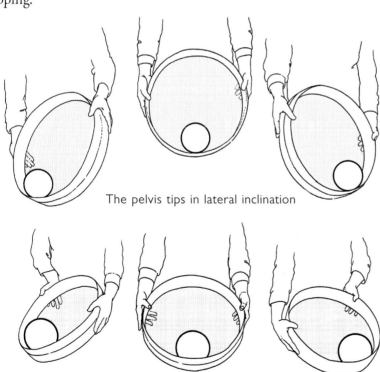

The pelvis tips in lateral inclination

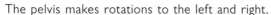

The pelvis makes rotations to the left and right.

PELVIC MOVEMENTS
WITH A LARGE RANGE OF MOTION

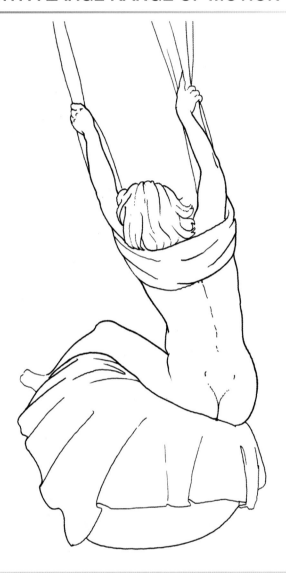

Up until now in this chapter we've looked at the pelvis as a solid piece. Now, in addition to movement at the hips to orient the internal space, we'll discuss movements that change the form of that internal space.

What Happens?

As we've seen, when the pelvic tilting movements are small, we concern ourselves with the fluidity of the movement, the comfort of the woman, and the rocking of the fetus. Here, the entire pelvis modifies its orientation.

If we increase the amplitude of the tilt, even by just one degree, we get a very different effect: this puts the muscles and ligaments of the hips under tension, which pulls on the three large pelvic bones. This intrinsic mobilization of the pelvis transforms the pelvic cavity: the iliac bones are pulled into different positions in relationship to each other and to the sacrum.

The innominate line, the ischial spines, and the pubic symphysis move around the femur heads.

Attention

Amplified tilting of the pelvis is indeed a movement of the pelvis and not a movement of the waist or the ribs. It is the pelvis that moves itself at the hips. This is an important bit of information, because it is very easy for the movement to shift to a different level.

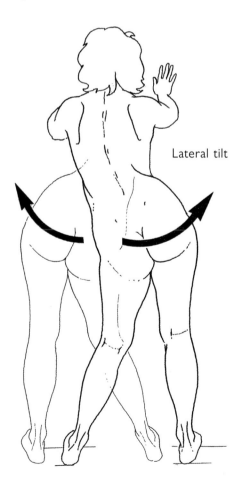

Lateral tilt

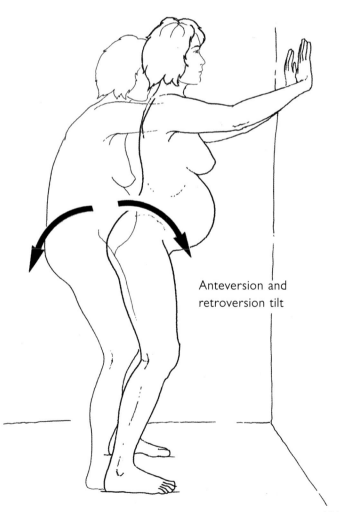

Anteversion and retroversion tilt

Transitions with Increased Amplitude

What Happens?

With transitions in a greater range, the intrinsic movements come more rapidly and the effects are stronger.

In Lateral Transition

- On the side making the movement, the hip abductors are put under tension. They pull the iliac bone into abduction, which moves the innominate line a little to the outside, enlarging the superior opening by a few millimeters on this side. A few millimeters may sound insignificant, but just that much can facilitate the passage of the fetus or the turning of its head at the passage from the first plane to the second plane.

- On the opposite side, if the leg is open enough (enough abduction), the hip adductors are put under tension, in partic-

ular the adductor magnus, which pulls the ischium and ischial spine outward. This is important for passage of the fetus from the third plane, just before the expulsion phase.

In Transition to the Back

The hamstrings are put under tension, pulling the ischia forward and bringing the iliac bones into retroversion. This helps guide the fetus to the posterior perineum.

In Transition to the Front

The hip flexors are put under tension. This pulls the iliac bones into anteversion/contra-nutation, which increases the distance between the sacral promontory and retropubic space and can facilitate passage of the fetus through the first and second planes.

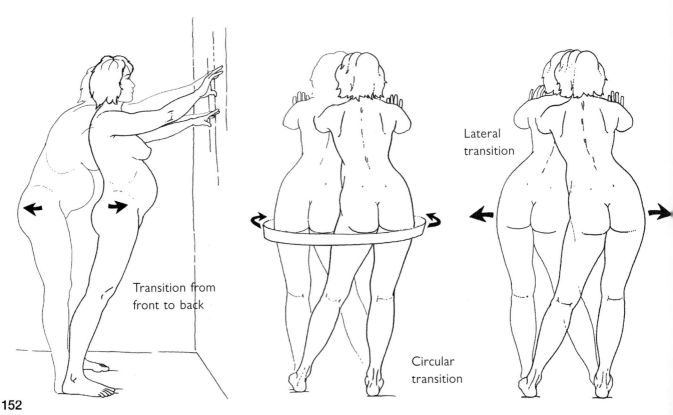

Transition from front to back

Circular transition

Lateral transition

Asymmetries Starting with the Lower Limbs

What Happens?

We have seen what the pelvis can do at the hips with the hips, knees, and ankles slightly bent and the legs more or less parallel.

- **When hip flexion is greater than 90°**, the posterior ligaments and the extensor muscles pull the iliac into nutation.
- **When hip extension is greater than 10°**, the iliac is pulled into contranutation.
- **When internal rotation is stressed**, the iliac is pulled into pronation and internal rotation.
- **When external rotation is stressed**, the iliac is pulled into supination and external rotation (see chapter 5).

Positioning the lower limbs asymmetrically influences and transforms the pelvis even more. When the woman is standing, sitting, or on all fours with her legs asymmetrical, the three openings become asymmetrical and:

- The two crests of the innominate line are no longer at the same height.
- The two ischial spines are no longer parallel in the frontal plane.
- The two pubic rami pull away from each other asymmetrically.
- The pubic symphysis is twisted (see p. 22).

The pelvis can transition and tilt on the lower limbs asymmetrically at the same time.

With what we have described so far, we can get an idea of the richness of movement at the pelvis and how these movements can facilitate the passage of the fetus through the birth canal.

The woman can combine these movements at all stages of delivery. When she moves her pelvis on the femur heads by making small swinging and circling motions, she uses the "sieve" effect to orient the baby and help it slip through the passage (see p. 149). Similarly, when she makes large movements with the pelvis, with her legs positioned asymmetrically, and changing from time to time the direction of the movement (for example, moving sometimes to the right and sometimes to the left), she transforms the birth canal to make room for the baby.

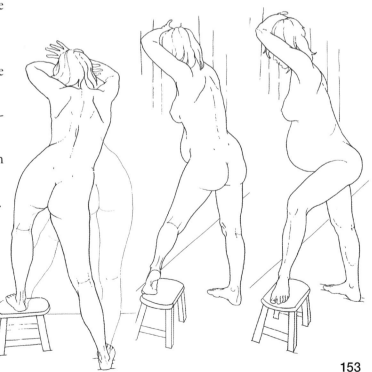

8

THE THREE
STAR POSITIONS

Standing, Sitting, Kneeling

Presentation

This chapter is dedicated to those of you who are at the point of giving birth, who want to better understand your body in this special moment of your life and to usher your infant into the world. We've tried to make the text less technical for two reasons.

- To give you ideas and tools to have with you at the time of delivery
- To make it possible for you to use these ideas during your pregnancy, in your daily life, or in preparation for childbirth

Why the "Three Star Positions"?
All the positions analyzed in chapter 6 serve to ease pain and facilitate the passage of the fetus through the birth canal. Among those positions, three offer the greatest possibilities for practice before the actual delivery.

- Standing, with the knees slightly bent (see p. 135)
- Sitting on a large ball (see p. 128)
- Kneeling/on all fours (see p. 129)

Here we envision these positions not as static but as real sources of movement. Each of these positions has its own characteristics. But each one can be transformed, changed, and adapted, so that it is easy to forget the original position. This is what makes these positions special and unique.

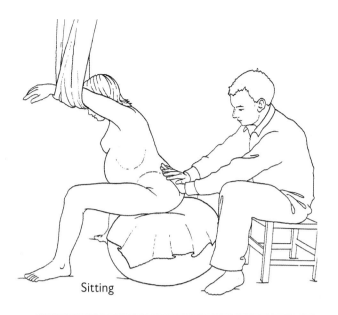

Sitting

These positions become "attitudes" in the sense that the woman is active, an active participant, rather than a spectator, at the birth. The staffs of obstetrics wards report that they often see women adopt these positions spontaneously, without being instructed to. They are used in numerous cultures, including ours, when the woman is listening to her body. Instinctively, she looks to work with the contractions to accommodate the passage of the baby. She starts to move or position herself in ways that feel right—silently or while making very individual sounds until the end of the contraction. It is for this reason that in the "Pelvis and Childbirth" workshops obstetrics personnel call these the **"star" positions.**

What Do the Three Positions Have in Common?

1. They are the positions in which the pelvis is the most free.

Without a doubt, the three star positions are those in which the pelvis is most free to move

on the legs (see "Unrestricted pelvis," p. 41).

Each woman can find the position that best suits her, and often that one factor is enough to ease the pain of a contraction. You can orient the three openings in a multidirectional fashion, with a wealth of variations and subtlety. You can enhance the connection between yourself and your baby.

2. You have a choice of leg positions.
You can move your legs in all directions. The bigger the movement, the more effect it has on your pelvis. You can change the position of each leg as you need to, without feeling obliged to stay on the same one. Another important point is that you find these positions intuitively: if you let it, the body can find the position that suits it best.

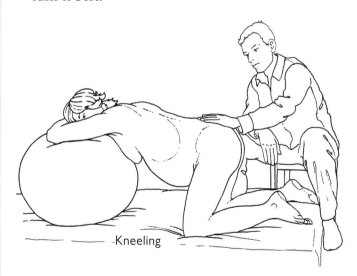

Kneeling

3. The sacrum is free and available.
The sacrum is free to move, which is necessary for the passage of the fetal head. The sacrum can recede, pulled by ligaments. And the three positions allow for access to the sacrum so that you can move your pelvis gently and at the same time have someone heat the sacrum with their

hands or massage it to relieve some of the tension on the sacroiliac ligaments.

4. Your hands are free to assist in mobilizing the pelvis.

Your hands are free so that you can support yourself at the edge of the bed, hang from a sling, or hold someone else's hands. You can use them to exert pressure to an area that needs it. And placed on the belly, they can support it, soothe it, and put you in contact with your baby.

5. You can support and suspend yourself.

You can choose the position of your trunk, arms, and head. The goal is to find the most comfortable position. In fact, when you eliminate the weight of your head (4 to 5 kg), arms (3 kg each), and trunk (thoracic rib cage/spine/viscera totaling about 30 kg) from the pelvis and the uterus, the abdominal muscles do not need to be recruited to hold the position. Therefore, in these positions most women feel less pressure on the working areas and more relief during uterine contractions.

6. Someone else's hands can assist.

The three positions allow for access to the low back and the sacroiliac joints. Heat from someone's hands or hot compresses will help relax the tissues in that area. Some women ask for strong pressure that they themselves cannot apply. In these positions, someone else can assist. The assistant can place his or her hands on either side of the pelvis, on the sacrum, or on the lower back, following the movements. The hands can support, accompany, and give a feeling of security, following attentively and respectfully the move-

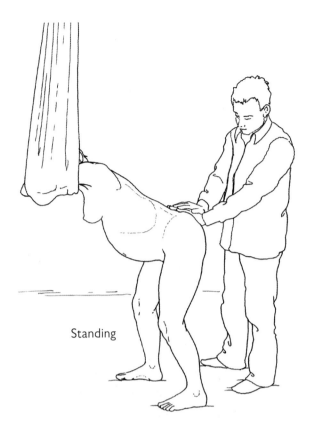

Standing

ments of the pelvis. This support requires that the person accompanying the woman be totally available and sincere and that he or she have a knowledge of where to put his or her hands.

This contact can help you better feel your pelvis and may allow you to stay "on the inside" with your baby in a more intimate way.

> "A husband explained that he felt more useful than he did with the birth of the first child thanks to all that he had learned about the positions and massage, knowing where to put his hands and why."
>
> THERESA MARTINEZ, MIDWIFE,
> ALACANT HEALTH CENTER, VALENCIA (SPAIN)

Standing Positions

Upright on the Feet

Initially it is important to feel how your feet are positioned on the floor. Can you feel how they make contact? Can you trust the floor to support you? This will give you more security as well as strength. The better your legs are situated, the more liberated your trunk is and the freer your pelvis.

You can start with your feet and legs a little separated: this gives you a wider base to support the weight of your body. Then, simply move your pelvis as if you were rocking your baby, and allow yourself to be carried by the movement. You can try to do this asymmetrically, as in the drawings below. Make the movements that please you, like a game, knowing that at the time of delivery you may or may not use them, but you'll find others that suit you better.

Suggestions and Variations

Standing, you can walk, sway, and swing your pelvis. You're putting the "sieve" effect into play

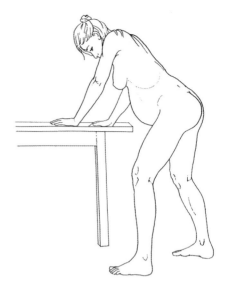

(see p. 149). You can discharge the weight of your trunk by leaning on a windowsill, the edge of a bed, a wall, or someone who is there to assist you.

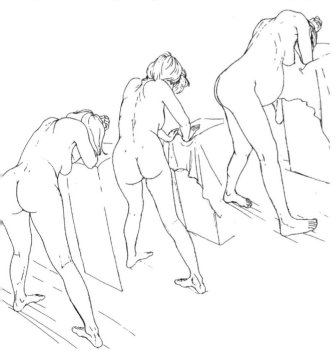

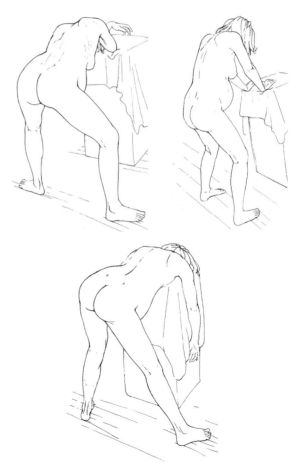

157

Suspended

Here we need to highlight the importance of this type of suspension and what makes it an interesting option for optimizing numerous movements described in this book. Suspension relieves the pelvis of the weight of the trunk so that it is much more available to move and is more free in its movement.

You can suspend yourself from a sling that is attached to the ceiling. Your arms are supported by the fabric and are relaxed. Your head can rest on your arms, and your feet are well situated on the floor. The weight of the pelvis on the femur heads is lessened. You can rock your baby by swinging your pelvis.

- Small circles: you orient it.
- Large circles, on one leg or the other: you create more space.
- Legs more or less separated, one turned in external rotation, the other in internal rotation: you favor its passage from one side or the other.

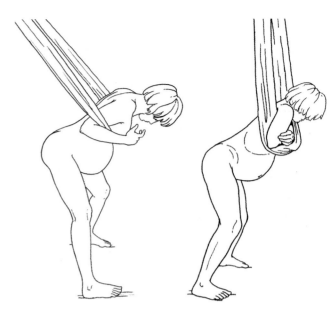

- One foot higher than the other (placed on a chair of stool), changing the leg positions according to how you feel: you allow the baby's head to adapt when it is turning.

All this is possible while just swinging the pelvis.

If you want contact or pressure on the sacrum, you can use your own hands for this, or ask someone assisting you.

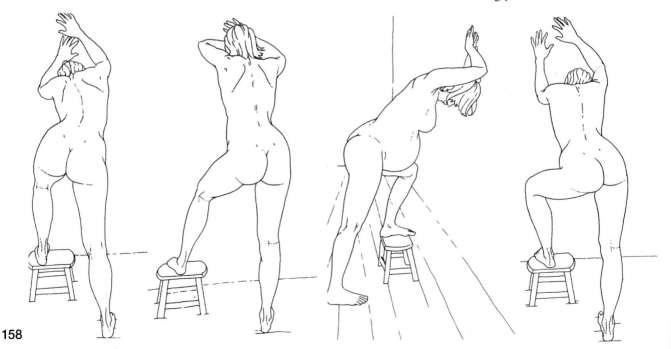

Sitting on a Large Ball

One of the best ways to move the pelvis is by sitting on a large ball. The ball is unstable, and so the pelvis is as well. Consequently, we are now finding balls in many maternity wards. Sitting on a ball is often recommended at the beginning of, and throughout, the dilation phase, with good results. There is a similarity between a ball that moves in all directions and the hip joints, which are also multidirectional. Combining this double mobility is a benefit for your delivery. If you are thinking about having an epidural, sitting on the ball can help you during the first part of the dilation phase. Without an epidural, it is a means to help you create the "sieve" effect (see p. 149) in later stages, while staying vertical so that you also work with gravity.

Things to Take into Account for Maximal Effect

1. The size of the ball must be proportional to your own size.

A person with short legs, sitting on a large ball, cannot place her feet securely on the floor. Conversely, a person with long legs, on a small ball, will sink into the ball so far that she will lose the ability to keep her pelvis free (see p. 41). Balls exist in many diameters, from 55 to 90 cm. Ideally there will be two or three sizes in the hospital. But to know what size best suits you, it is better to try them out before the day of your delivery.

2. Get used to the ball before your delivery date.

It is important before your delivery to get used to the feeling of instability on the ball, to find the position in which you feel the most secure, and to feel the pelvis move at the hips. You can explore specific actions.

- Sit far back on the ball and then move far forward, and move from one position to the other.
- Slide from one side to the other.
- Draw a circle with your pelvis, moving the ischia from right to left (remember to change direction, because we tend to always go in the same direction).

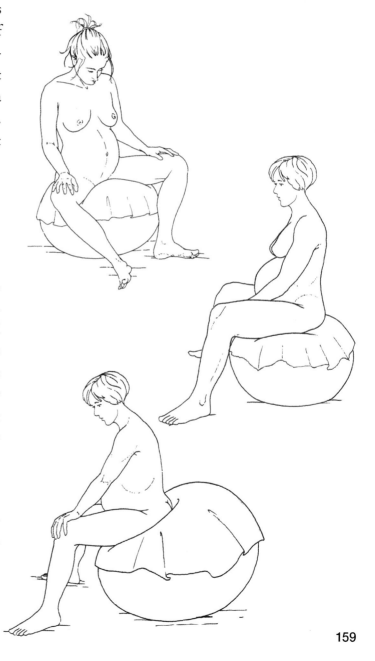

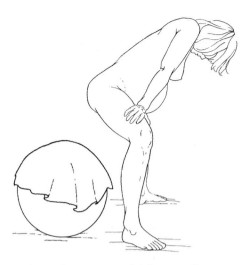

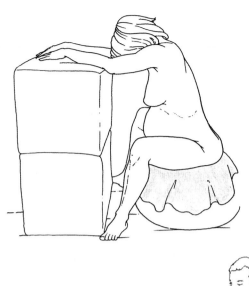

3. Explore the way in which your feet support you.

The first thing to learn is how to get on and off the ball. This may seem a bit banal, but it is a major cause of failure.

> **Step 1:** Before sitting down, feel how your trunk is supported on your legs, and feel the strength in them.
>
> **Step 2:** Slowly sit down on the ball, without losing the feeling of strength in your legs.
>
> **Step 3:** Feel when the weight of your trunk passes from your legs to the ball.
>
> **Step 4:** Do not at first lose contact with your feet on the floor or the sensation of the

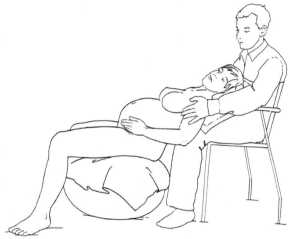

weight of your body on your feet when you are seated on the ball. After you've become comfortable, you can rest against someone who supports your back.

4. Find anchors and points of contact for your hands.

The first few times you use the ball, it is important to have something stationary in front of you. This can be a heavy chair, the edge of a bed, or another person. This way you are supported and can relax and explore the various ways of moving on the ball.

Later, your hands will find points of contact to use for pulling or pushing your body.

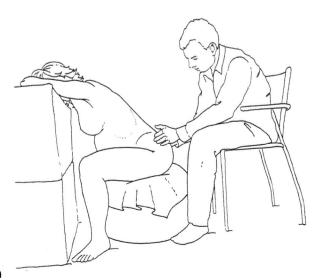

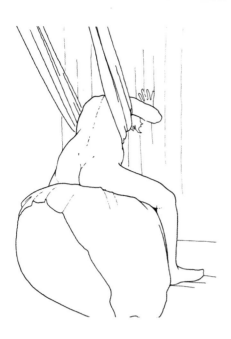

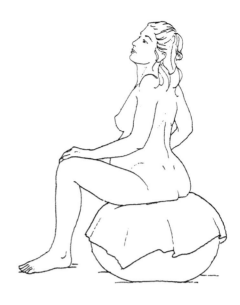

Try, too, putting pressure on your knees, which in turn sends pressure to your legs and to the floor, and discover how pushing with your hands can move the pelvis.

5. Move primarily from the hip joints.

Once you feel secure, start to move your pelvis from the hips. You can direct it in different directions. Make small circles, small figure eights, or fluid movements to produce the "sieve" effect (see p. 149). If you make the same movements larger, you change the shape of the birth canal (see chapter 7). These should

not be mechanical or learned movements; instead, seek out movements for the sensations they create. Trust how you feel. Your body will find the movements and directions it needs.

6. Position your legs asymmetrically for greater effect.

When you're comfortable with sitting on the ball, and only then, you can also move your legs. Stay alert and aware of the sensations so that you do not end up in a position that puts you off balance and causes you to tense up or to fall. You know now how to create asymmetries: internal and external rotation will move

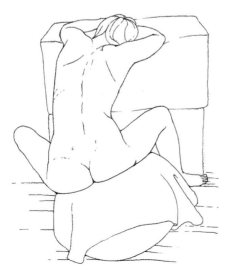

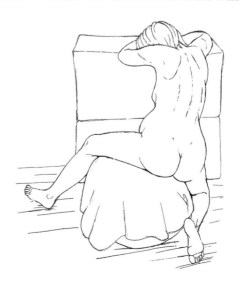

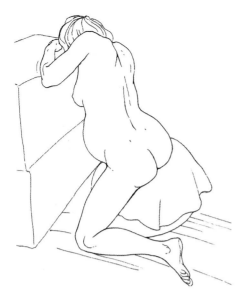

7. Suspend yourself from a sling attached to the ceiling.

This position has the same recommendations as for the upright position, but there is an advantage here: your legs and trunk are supported by the sling, and the pelvis is supported and rocked by the ball. It is also more relaxing.

The hook from which the sling will be suspended needs to be well anchored.

The sling offers you the interesting possibility of eliminating a large part of the weight of your trunk on your pelvis, while at the same time keeping the pelvis free and vertical. The sacrum is free from the weight of the trunk and is slightly pulled by the back muscles. You need to be confident of the security of the sling so that you can be rocked by its movement, let your head rest in the folds, and so forth.

Midwives who have proposed the sling to women say that they are very encouraged by the result. They say that women can usually stay a long time in this position and be more at ease, centered, and able to stay in contact with their bodies and their babies.

the iliac bones, as will bigger movements (see pp. 90–91).

You will feel the stretching and the tension at the inside of your hips and to the back, at the sacroiliac joint, as the iliac bones and the sacrum move in turn. Your birth canal becomes a transformable passageway. Again, be guided by what you feel, and your body will find what benefits it. You will no doubt feel how tension and pain are alleviated by the movement.

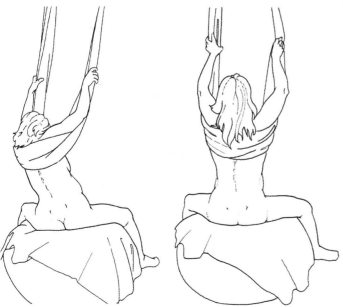

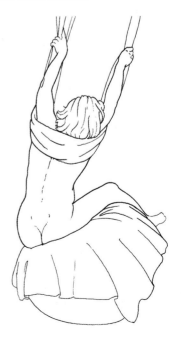

Kneeling Position/On All Fours

This position has already been analyzed on page 130. Here the pelvis is very free to move in all directions. The position of the hips favors a relaxation of the sacroiliac joints. The weight of the baby falls to the pubis and to the hammock of the abdomen, and the sacrum frees up.

For a long time this position was looked down on. Now it is accepted and even proposed in hospital settings.

How Do You Get Ready?

Get comfortable. Here are a few important notes:

- Place your knees on a soft support (pillows, foam, et cetera).

- Separate your legs slightly to create a wide base of support.
- Support the weight of the trunk more with your legs than your arms. Otherwise, your wrists will get tired very fast. Even better, put your trunk on a support.

Ina May Gaskin, the midwife who created the Gaskin maneuver, proposes this position of being on all fours in cases of asynclitism. We understand why many women use this position during the dilation phase and some, spontaneously, during the expulsion.

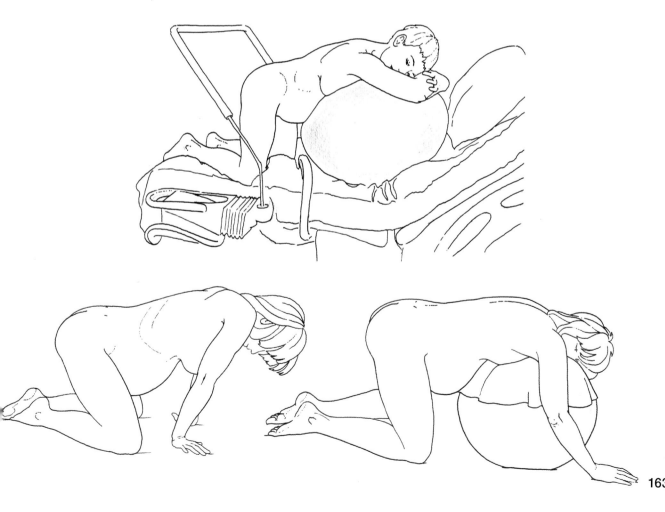

Several Kinds of Support

You can rest your trunk on a chair with a large pillow, on a firm or soft support, or on the legs of someone who is seated securely and can still move his or her legs while massaging your back. You can also rest your trunk on a raised bed or on a large ball, which can give at the same time support that is firm, soft, and mobile.

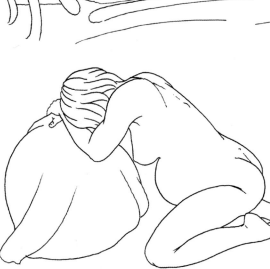

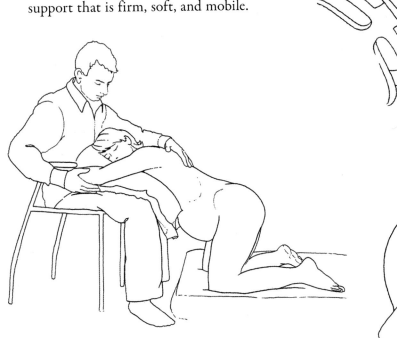

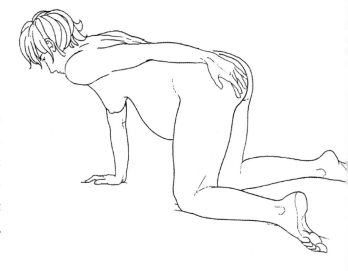

How Do We Move?

In this position, do you know how to find your ischia? Find them, one at a time, with the hand of the same side. Once you have found them, imagine that you have placed small lights on them. They will shine to the back. Now, slowly, tip the lights so that they illuminate the ceiling, return to your starting position, and then shine the lights on the floor. This image helps us use our hips rather than our back. The movement has to be initiated at the hip joints. Finally, imagine that the lights are going to shine all over. Let the movement travel up your spine to your head, knowing that it originated at the hips.

Position Your Legs Asymmetrically

Positioning your legs asymmetrically changes the shape of the inside of the pelvis. Kneeling, you can place your legs in various positions while keeping the weight of your trunk supported and the pelvis free to move. You can gently rotate one leg internally and the other externally, then change sides, while at the same time rocking your pelvis.

The important thing in all of these kneeling positions is that they help ease the pain.

On the day of delivery it is not certain that you will want to use these positions, but at least you will know them and have them at your disposal. If you have actually tried these movements your body memory will be able to recall them on the day of your delivery.

"I am fortunate to work in a hospital where women are at liberty to deliver as they want. Knowledge of pelvic movements helps me to understand why women 'squirm' in delivery and often adopt asymmetrical positions of the pelvis depending on the position of the fetus when it starts its descent into the birth canal.

"I've observed that many women resort to pelvic asymmetry, independent of the position (standing, on all fours, on the bed, on the table). Almost all finish with a leg a little more forward than the other and with several degrees of internal rotation of the femurs."

ASCENSION GOMEZ, MIDWIFE,
HUERCAL-OVERA HOSPITAL, ALMERIA (SPAIN)

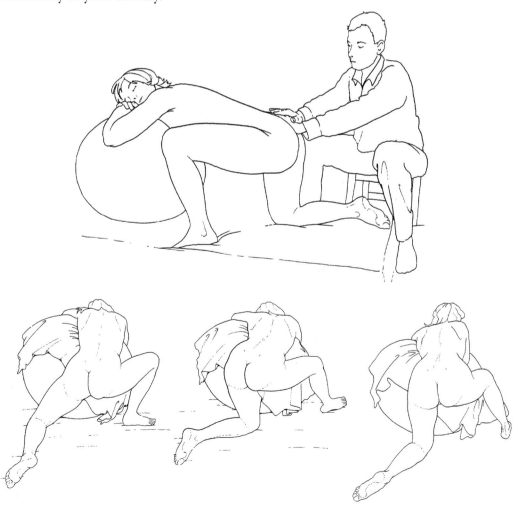

165

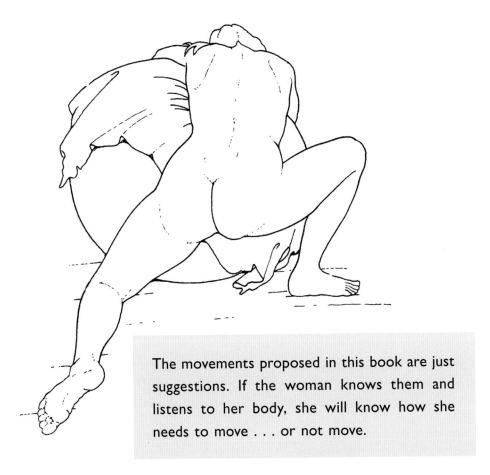

The movements proposed in this book are just suggestions. If the woman knows them and listens to her body, she will know how she needs to move . . . or not move.

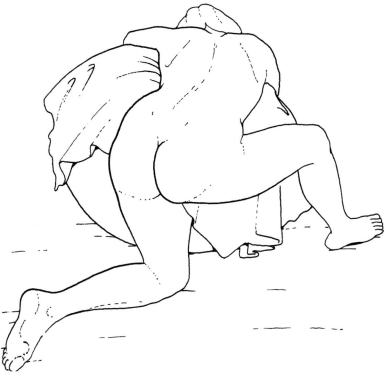

ANATOMY OF MOVEMENT CERTIFICATION PROGRAMS

The Blandine Calais-Germain Method

This approach to anatomy is multisensorial, including palpation of anatomical models, identification on your own body, and observation and creation of visuals, drawings, and representations of internal anatomy, alternated between equal amounts of theory and practice of specific movements. The certification programs are designed for health professionals, teachers of physical methodologies, and people who want to deepen their understanding of the body. For further information on these course offerings go to **www.calais-germain.com**.

"Anatomy and Preparation for Childbirth" Cycle

A. Pelvis, Movement, Delivery (about 30 hours)

A1. Mobility of the Pelvis in Childbirth (15 hours of courses)

Presentation of anatomy pertaining to intrinsic/extrinsic movements of the pelvis and consequences for the pelvic cavity. Presentation of a repertoire of movements and positions corresponding to the stages of childbirth.

A2. Analysis and Practice of Positions for Pelvic Mobility (15 hours of courses)

Experimentation and analysis of positions that women assume spontaneously when giving birth, or positions and movements that we propose that favor the passage of the baby through the birth canal while diminishing pain. How to use materials. The role of the companion.

B. Movement and Childbirth (about 30 hours of courses)

B1. The Breath during Childbirth (15 hours of courses)

Based on the books *Breathing* by Blandine Calais-Germain and *Conscience Sensorielle* by Charles Brooks. Presents the physiological movements of breathing using three parameters: flux, volume, and location. Anatomy: the skeleton when breathing and set in motion, the organs of respiration, and pulmonary elasticity. Muscles of inhalation and exhalation. Role and parameters of these structures at specific times during the delivery.

B2. Preparing Your Body during Pregnancy (15 hours of courses)
Starting with an anatomical analysis, we offer a base of physical practice to facilitate stability and/or mobility of the pelvis, improve postural adaptations to pregnancy, prevent back and pubic pain, and facilitate good breathing. Positions and movements are analyzed anatomically with the idea of creating a personalized series of connected movements for practice.

Professional Certification in Perineum and Movement

Prevention Exercises for the Pelvic Floor (90 hours of courses)
Perineum and Movement is a repertoire of movements that are commonly used to solicit the perineum with the goal of toning, relaxing, and making it more supple while also bringing more awareness to the area. The exercises are constantly changing three parameters: the action of gravity on the perineum, the stretching/shortening of the region, and the forces (hypotension, rhythmic pressure).

The "Perineum" workshop is a prerequisite for this workshop. It includes three complementary areas of instruction.

- **Anatomical makeup of the male and female perineum:** a study of the forces on the perineum as we play with movement
- **Practice repertoire:** 10-hour protocol
- **Methodology of teaching:** pedagogical practice sessions

Optionally, a competency test can be taken and a certificate issued that allows professionals to teach this method.

Useful Practitioner Tools

"The Pelvis Moves and Transforms" Notebooks
The method described in chapter 7 is covered in detail for professionals. Available soon at www.calais-germain.com.

Four Instruction Binders

Collections of illustrations by Blandine Calais-Germain designed for teaching about pregnancy and preparation for childbirth. Four different notebooks of twenty-five pedagogical illustrations, for specific teaching programs.

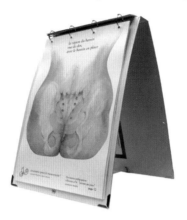

- Movements for childbirth
- The female perineum and preparation for childbirth
- The female perineum (perineum and movement)
- Understanding your pelvis for childbirth

The Mobile Pelvis

A special collection designed for explaining and illustrating the intrinsic movements of the pelvis described in chapter 3 of this book. Can be held easily in the hands while demonstrating pelvic movements. For midwives, physical therapists, and movement professionals who prepare women for childbirth. On sale at www.calais-germain.com.

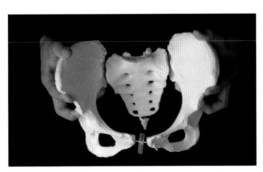

BIBLIOGRAPHY

Other Books by Blandine Calais-Germain

Anatomy of Breathing. Seattle: Eastlake Press, 2006.

Anatomy of Movement. Seattle: Eastlake Press, 2007.

Anatomy of Movement Exercises. Seattle: Eastlake Press, 2008.

The Female Pelvis. Seattle: Eastlake Press, 2003.

No-Risk Abs. Rochester, Vt.: Healing Arts Press, 2011.

Anatomy

Basmajian, P. V. *Anatomie.* Paris: Librairie Maloine, n.d.

Bouchet, A., and J. Cuilleret. *Anatomie topographique, descriptive et fonctionnelle.* Paris: SIMEP Éditions, 1991.

Kahle, W., H. Leonhard, and W. Platze. *Anatomie.* Paris: Flammarion, 1986.

Kapandji, A. *Physiologie articulaire* 1, 2, 3. Paris: Librairie Maloine, 1999.

Sobotta. *Atlas d'anatomie humaine.* Paris: Librairie Maloine, 1977.

Vandervael, F. *Analyse des mouvements du corps humain.* Paris: Librairie Maloine/ éd. Desoer, n.d.

Vigué, Martin. *Grand Atlas d'anatomie humaine.* Paris: Désiris, 2006.

Other Books on Childbirthing

Barbira Freedman, Françoise, and Doriel Hall. *Prenatal Yoga for Conception, Pregnancy, and Birth.* London: Lorenz Books, 2002.

Gaskin, Ina May. *Guide to Childbirth.* New York: Bantam Books, 2003.

———. *Parteria Espiritual.* Argentina: Mujer Sabia Editores, 2007.

Gasquet, (de) B. *Bien-être et maternité.* Paris: Implexe Éditions du Seuil, 1996.

Odent, Michael. *Genèse de l'homme écologique.* Paris: Épi, 1979.

———. *Histoires de naissances.* Paris: Épi, 1985.

———. *Votre bébé est le plus beau des mammifieres.* Paris: Albin Michel, 1990.

Simkin, P., and R. Ancheta. *The Labor Progress Handbook: Early Interventions to Prevent and Treat Dystocia.* Oxford: Blackwell Publishing, 2005.

Journals

"Hors série Naître aujourd'hui." *Générations Tao,* no. 5 (2006).

"Périnée et maternité. Les Dossiers de l'Obstétrique collection. Grand sujets," *Éditions* E.L. P.E.A. (1999).

Articles

Bruner J. P., S. B. Drummond, A. L. Meenan, and Ina May Gaskin. All-fours maneuver for reducing shoulder dystocia during labor. *Journal of Reproductive Medicine* (May 1998).

Fenwick, L., and P. Simkin. Maternal positioning to prevent or alleviate dystocia in labor. *Clinical Obstetrics and Gynaecology* 30, no. 1 (1987): 83–89.

Videos

Positions for Childbirth, by the physical therapy department of Adelaide Hospital, South Australia, www.foundationstudios.com.au.

Pour que ses jours fleurissent, a film by Nicole Ferry, ferry.nicole@gmail.com.

INDEX

pronation of the iliac, 60, 61, 62, 92, 106–7, 116, 142, 153
    defined, 41
pubic symphysis, 7, 12, 18, 22–24
    effect of movement on, 56–62, 151, 153

reclining. *See under* birthing positions
restricted pelvis. *See* pressure, application of
retroversion, 29, 48, 70, 76–77, 94, 149
    birthing chair and, 99
    fetus and, 147
    in semi-reclining position, 113
    See also anteversion; lateroversion; sieve effect

sacrococcyx, 15
sacroiliac joint, 19–21, 162
    opening of, 62
    pain relief and, 118, 137, 138
    See also ligaments
sacrolumbar joint, 25–26
sacrolumbar region,15
sacrum, 14–16
    connection to iliac bone, 8
    contranutation of, 50–51, 58, 85, 98, 105, 107
    innominate lines, 16, 19 (*See also* innominate lines)
    location of, 3, 14
    mobility of, 111, 155–56 (*See also* star positions)
    nutation of, 46–47, 83, 85, 114–15
    pressure on, 98–99, 105
    promontory, 16, 34
    sacral plateau, 16
    sacral wing, 16, 34
    three parts of, 15
    See also sacroiliac joint
sagittal plane, 43
    movements of, 45–53
Santamaria, Pepa, 105

sieve effect, 102, 130, 134, 153, 157, 159, 161
    defined, 149
Sims position, 124
sitting. *See* birthing positions
sling. *See* suspension
slip, 41
slip effect, 149
spine
    pelvis connected to, 3, 18, 25–26, 67, 83–84
squatting. *See* birthing positions
stages of childbirth. *See* childbirth, four stages of
standing. *See* birthing positions
star positions, 154–66. *See also* birthing positions
superior opening of pelvis, 34
    asymmetrical, 122
    closing, 85, 94
    enlarging, 50, 52, 56, 63, 89, 93, 96, 98, 100
supination of the iliac, 60, 61, 93, 100, 153
    defined, 41
suspension, 136–43, 158
synovial fluid, 19

table. *See* birthing table
thighs, 30–31
threading effect, 102
transverse plane, 43
    movements in, 54, 58–60
transversospinalis muscles, 85
trochanter, 27, 30
    effect of movement on, 101
    pressure on, 101
trunk, 29

unrestricted pelvis positions, 41, 68–69

varicose veins, 143
vulva, 7

Books of Related Interest

Gentle Birth Choices
By Barbara Harper, R.N.
Photographs by Suzanne Arms

Vaccinations: A Thoughtful Parent's Guide
How to Make Safe, Sensible Decisions about the Risks, Benefits, and Alternatives
by Aviva Jill Romm

Natural Health after Birth
The Complete Guide to Postpartum Wellness
by Aviva Jill Romm

Birth without Violence
by Frédérick Leboyer, M.D.

The Art of Giving Birth
With Chanting, Breathing, and Movement
by Frédérick Leboyer, M.D.

Natural Mothering
A Guide to Holistic Therapies for Pregnancy, Birth, and Early Childhood
by Nicky Wesson

The Art of Conscious Parenting
The Natural Way to Give Birth, Bond with, and Raise Healthy Children
by Jeffrey L. Fine, Ph.D., with Dalit Fine, M.S.

Celebrating the Great Mother
A Handbook of Earth-Honoring Activities for Parents and Children
by Cait Johnson and Maura D. Shaw

INNER TRADITIONS • BEAR & COMPANY
P.O. Box 388
Rochester, VT 05767
1-800-246-8648
www.InnerTraditions.com

Or contact your local bookseller